THE COMPLETE BOOK OF
NAUTILUS® TRAINING

Michael D. Wolf, Ph.D.

CONTEMPORARY
BOOKS, INC.
CHICAGO

Library of Congress Cataloging in Publication Data

Wolf, Michael D.
   The complete book of Nautilus training.

   Includes index.
   1. Weight lifting.   2. Weight lifting—Equipment and
supplies.   3. Physical fitness.   I. Title.
GV546.W635   1984   613.7'1   83-27310
ISBN 0-8092-5455-7

All photographs © 1984 by Marti Cohen Wolf.

All artwork by Vanessa Hill.

CONTENTS

ACKNOWLEDGMENTS

Special thanks to the people behind the scenes, in front of the camera, and, most of all, behind the camera:

My ace photographer (and wonderful wife), Marti.

My editor, Nancy Crossman.

My models: Brenda Bernhardt Frasca, Major Steve Butcher, Jerry Conklin, and Jan Stritzler.

Richie Orenstein of Club Meadowlands in Secaucus, New Jersey, where most of the photos were taken.

Risa Friedman of New York's One-to-One Center for Movement and Fitness, and Gregory Cilek of the Manhattan Plaza Health Club, who were also gracious in extending their facilities for photography.

Our ever-so-capable photographic assistants Mom and Dad Wolf and Jon Coron.

You are all very sincerely appreciated.

INTRODUCTION: *ANOTHER* NAUTILUS BOOK?

You've read every book on Nautilus training, so why read another? Give me a minute before you put this book down. This is *it*. This is complete. The works. The whole show. The real thing. The whole ball of wax.

What I've tried to do is put enough information in one place, in *easily* understood form, with loads of photos and drawings, to make *you* one of the "experts."

You ask, "Aren't there enough exercise experts already?" My answer is that you would run out of experts before you ran out of fingers and toes to count them on. There's a serious misinformation problem in the exercise field today, and most of the "experts" have a poor knowledge of anatomy, physiology, and biomechanics (the physics of body movement). A majority of them base their understanding of exercise equipment on three-sentence, one-photo instruction manuals. Though I'm seeing more and more exceptions these days, my travels for Nautilus have brought me into constant contact with self-proclaimed experts who couldn't fill a thimble with what they "know" about exercise or Nautilus.

I want to make *you* an expert. It's easier than you think. It won't require a great deal of work or time. You will, of course, have to buy this book. What will you get for your investment? Answers to the following questions and more:

- What is "fitness"? What are the components that add up to make you fit? Where does Nautilus come in? Does it do it all? (To this latter, no.)
- How does your body work? Why do you absolutely, positively *have* to understand the aerobic and anaerobic systems to train correctly? Muscle . . . what types are there? How are they controlled? Does this affect your training? How does muscle grow?
- What's the truth about nutrition and exercise? Nutrition and weight control? Is it true that the average person can save enough money by forgetting about vitamin, mineral, and protein supplements to take a month-long vacation in Hawaii?

- The Nautilus Operating Manual: How do the machines work? *Do* the machines work? (Yes.) How does the beginner use each of the machines? The advanced trainee? What kinds of workouts can be cooked up?
- Aerobic exercise: Where does it fit in? What are your aerobic choices? How are they performed? How can you add them to your training plans?
- Starting and finishing: How do you warm up? Stretch? Cool down?

Let's assume you take the giant step and purchase this book. Let's even assume you go beyond that and actually read it. What does becoming an expert do for you?

It will let you plan an intelligent approach to total health care through exercise and nutrition. It will reduce your injury risk and improve results from your Nautilus and aerobic training. It will probably make you the envy of everyone at your fitness center. And, most importantly, it will make you an intelligent consumer, less likely to contribute to the tens of billions of dollars Americans waste each year on needless nutritional supplements and out-for-a-buck fitness centers.

The Greeks said it first, and it's my goal for you through this book: *Mens sana in corpore sano*—A sound mind in a sound body. I hope you enjoy, and *use*, this book.

1
NAUTILUS AND THE COMPONENTS OF FITNESS

Of all the phrases that have been used to describe Nautilus, the most accurate is "time-efficient fitness." If you're looking for a good, hard, five-hour workout, you've definitely come to the wrong place! On the other hand, many of the claims that have been made by and about Nautilus are a bit overstated. It won't do all things for all people in sixty minutes a week.

What *can* Nautilus do? How does it fit into the overall fitness framework? What activities must supplement your Nautilus training to make you optimally fit?

THE COMPONENTS OF FITNESS

Since we should establish just what fitness is before analyzing the Nautilus contribution, let's look at its nine major components:

- Muscular strength
- Muscular endurance
- Cardiovascular or aerobic endurance
- Anaerobic power
- Speed
- Agility
- Flexibility
- Balance
- Neuromuscular (motor) coordination

What can you expect from Nautilus in regard to these components?

Strength

Strength is the ability to create force in one maximal effort. You didn't need this book to tell you that this is the primary contribution of Nautilus to total fitness. Given proper form and sufficient intensity, the average individual (male or female) will see strength gains of 2%–5% per week. Some muscles will respond quickly, some slowly, and some not at all (it's genetic), but you'll be very pleasantly surprised at the time efficiency of Nautilus training. One set on each machine, taken to momentary muscular failure, turns the trick.

Expect a lightning fast workout, performed in an empty fitness center with seat heights and weights set beforehand, to take you eighteen minutes. In a crowded center, this time may extend out to forty-five minutes or more. This may reduce the anaerobic benefits of training, but can actually increase your strength gains. But I'm getting ahead of myself. More on that later.

Muscular Endurance

Muscular Endurance is the ability to maintain a submaximal muscular force for a prolonged period of time. It's still mostly guesswork here because the research has been poor and incomplete. From my experience with elite athletes in about ten different sports, I would say that Nautilus circuit training (moving rapidly from machine to machine) has a strong, positive effect on muscular endurance.

Cardiovascular/ Aerobic Endurance

Cardiovascular/Aerobic Endurance is the ability to work for extended periods of time at a relatively high proportion of one's maximal oxygen-processing capacity. You'll learn just what this means in the next chapter, but for now, think of a marathon runner as the best example of aerobic endurance. It's going to take several pages in the next chapter to convince you of this, but Nautilus—despite its ability to keep your heart rate sky-high for 30 minutes—is not more than 60% aerobic. (This means that 40% of the energy for Nautilus training is coming from "anaerobic" sources.) Since exercise must be at least 65%–70% aerobic before you see any changes in your cardiovascular system, you'll need to add aerobic exercise(s) to your overall workout strategy.

In fact, research has shown that Nautilus training becomes less and less aerobic as you increase in fitness. Several studies have noted that trained athletes are as much as 65% anaerobic during high intensity Nautilus training! Chapter 11 is your complete guide to aerobic exercise, giving you the lowdown on aerobic choices, how they're performed, and how they can be fitted into your workout plans.

Anaerobic Power

Anaerobic Power is the ability to create high amounts of work (force over a distance) in a short amount of time. That speaks very well for Nautilus here! If your fitness center has enough slack time to allow those 18-minute, super Nautilus circuit workouts, you'll experience tremendous anaerobic benefits. Some of the older Nautilus literature speaks mysteriously of a "metabolic effect." It's very likely that anaerobic power is what they were talking about. The best example of anaerobic power is the 400-meter trackman who must provide all the energy for his sprinting from his anaerobic system.

Speed

Speed is the ability to move a body part, or the entire body, at high velocities. This ability is dependent on the components of both strength and anaerobic power. You should be prepared to hear several different stories about strength training and speed. For now, let me state that researchers closed the case about 30 years ago, showing conclusively that slow-speed, high-intensity strength work improved the speed of muscle contraction. For some reason, though, barbell advocates and some old-time football coaches have been spreading rumors that slow weight training leads to slow movement. Don't believe it. There's strong evidence from nearly every sport that slow, high-intensity strength work improves speed. As we'll see later, the alternative explosive training methods advocated by some are five times as dangerous and not nearly as productive.

Flexibility

Flexibility is the capacity of muscles to remain pliable in conforming to new configurations. The good news: most Nautilus machines effectively place you in stretched starting positions, preventing the usual reduction in your "range of motion." The bad news: permanent increases in flexibility occur *only* when a warmed muscle is held in a stretched position for at least 20 or 30 seconds. Nautilus *will* keep you from getting muscle-bound. It *won't* handle the weekend (or weekday) athlete's flexibility needs. Those will be taken care of in Chapter 12.

Balance and Agility

Balance and Agility are abilities that allow the body to remain stable and poised in spite of threatening forces. With little or no research to refer to, we're left with common sense here. I would bet that Nautilus has a significant effect on agility, because it's determined by many of the components mentioned above. I wouldn't even venture a guess about effects on balance. If your sport requires either or both of these components, the best way to improve them is through actual performance of the sport skills. Skip those generally silly agility drills you see in

magazines or on television—no one has ever proved they work.

Neuromuscular Coordination

Neuromuscular (motor) Coordination is the ability to make your muscles do what your brain tells them to do. Strength training definitely improves your brain's ability to use muscle for strength work, but we're not so clear about the general effects on motor coordination. Your best bet for improving this component is, again, actual performance of your sport skills. There's no substitute for good practice!

Where does that leave us? Nautilus can't do it all in sixty minutes a week, but it *can* be the cornerstone of a total fitness program. With an equal time expenditure on aerobic exercise, and some attention to warm-ups and flexibility exercise, you're going to have a blast watching your entire life change.

2
YOUR OPERATING MANUAL: RUNNING THE ENGINES

The first step in becoming a fitness expert is learning about energy. In the human body, it all boils down to one little compound: ATP, or *adenosine triphosphate*. ATP is the fuel for all bodily functions, from thought to movement to digestion. Given some background on where it comes from, and where it goes, you'll be well on your way toward an understanding of training physiology. And won't it be nice to figure out your own training programs!

ATP—THE CURRENCY OF ENERGY

Adenosine triphosphate is a tiny storehouse of energy. It is made up of three "phosphate" groups (phosphorous and oxygen) bound to one adenosine molecule. Should one of the phosphate groups be broken off the ATP molecule to leave *ADP*, or adenosine *di*phosphate, a great deal of energy is released. It is this energy which is put to use by the body. ADP is not broken down further in muscle (to *AMP*, or adenosine *monophosphate*), but this does occur elsewhere in the body.

At the beginning of exercise, the ATP stores in the entire body only add up to about three ounces, or enough to keep any muscle working for about three seconds. Should a muscle be asked to work for more than three seconds, there must be a new and fast source of ATP. Fulfilling this role is another chemical compound called *creatine phosphate*, or CP. Watch this neat trick: when CP is broken down into creatine and phosphate, the energy released can take an ADP molecule, tack on a loose phosphate, and create a new ATP molecule. There is enough CP stored in the average body to keep your muscles bathed in ATP for up to ten seconds. One hundred meter sprinters are examples of athletes who depend upon this ATP–CP system. Weightlifters and powerlifters may compete solely with stored ATP.

4

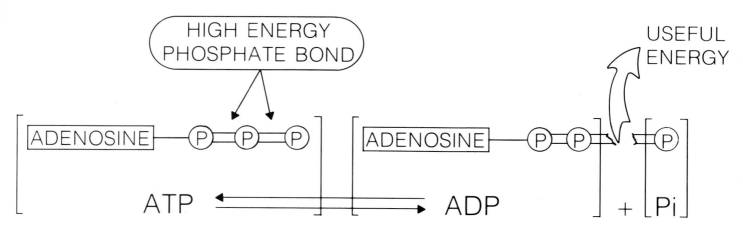

When adenosine triphosphate is broken down to adenosine diphosphate, the energy released can be used in the muscle contraction process.

ANAEROBIC AND AEROBIC PROCESSING

The story gets a little bit more complicated if exercise lasts beyond ten seconds. For about the next 60 seconds of work by a particular muscle, energy will be largely derived from your anaerobic system, the one that burns only carbohydrates and doesn't need oxygen. At about the two-minute mark, the aerobic system, which uses oxygen to burn carbos, fats, and proteins, is about 50% active. A specific muscle must be contracting for at least five to seven minutes before its aerobic machinery is running at full tilt.

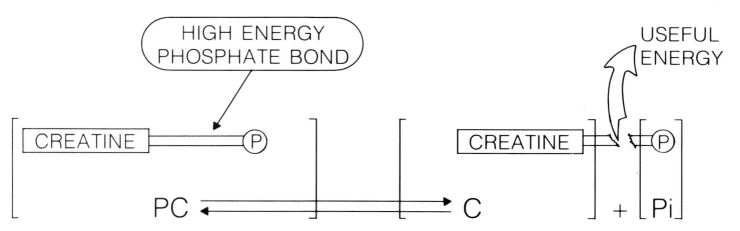

The energy released from creatine phosphate (or phosphocreatine) breakdown is used to rebuild ATP from ADP plus free phosphate. Phosphocreatine can later be rebuilt from creatine and free phosphate.

To Each Its Own

Notice how I keep writing about anaerobic and aerobic systems *within* specific muscles? There is *not* one centrally-located organ, like the heart, called the aerobic system. Each muscle in the body has its own aerobic and anaerobic systems. As we'll see in a moment, this is the reason why Nautilus training, though it may last 30 minutes and keep your heart rate high, is not an aerobic exercise.

AEROBIC/ANAEROBIC CONTRIBUTIONS TO EXERCISE

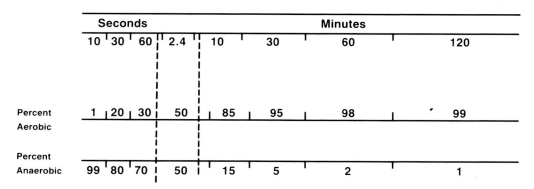

	Seconds				Minutes			
	10 30 60	2.4	10	30	60		120	
Percent Aerobic	1 20 30	50	85	95	98		99	
Percent Anaerobic	99 80 70	50	15	5	2		1	

Exercise lasting less than a minute is between 70% and 99% anaerobic. The aerobic system warms up slowly, and is bearing only 50% of the ATP production duties at two minutes.

Carbohydrates and Anaerobics

Asking a human being to live on a low-carbohydrate diet is about as smart as getting a blood transfusion from a stone. Here are just a few of the reasons why:

- Carbohydrates are the *only* fuel for anaerobic metabolism, which is responsible for 50% of the first two minutes of exercise.
- It takes the body 20–30 minutes (or more) of exercise to begin the breakdown of fat for energy. If carbohydrate stores are low, the body will turn to protein first and start breaking down muscles and organs.
- Fat doesn't become the major supplier of energy for muscle until exercise has lasted 45 minutes to an hour or more. Up to this point, the preferred fuel is carbohydrates.
- One of the small compounds that results from the breakdown of carbohydrates is essential for normal *fat* metabolism.
- The brain can *only* use glucose (a simple carbohydrate) for fuel.

As you'll learn later in Chapter 4 (Feeding the Machine), your diet should contain at least 60% carbohydrates.

We've so far established that the first ten seconds of exercise require no food sources whatsoever, using stored ATP and CP. The anaerobic system, with carbohydrates as the major fuel source, takes over at this point and provides ATP for another 60–90 seconds. (The aerobic system gradually enters the picture as time passes.) Let's look at the anaerobic process more closely.

Whether the carbohydrate is found in a simple form such as table sugar, or in a complex form such as a potato, it must be broken down to glucose before the anaerobic system can do its thing. There has been much publicity recently about fructose, since it is treated differently than glucose when metabolized. At the time this was written, however, there was little evidence that fructose had any special effects on exercise.

Once the digestive process has reduced the carbohydrates to glucose, the anaerobic enzymes go to work on further breakdown of the sugar. In the act of taking one glucose and changing it into a simpler compound called *pyruvic acid,* two molecules of ATP are formed. It is these ATPs that muscle can use for contraction during the first two minutes of exercise, but you haven't seen anything yet. The aerobic system, if it gets the chance, can take that pyruvic acid molecule and wring another 36 ATPs out of it.

AEROBICS—WHAT IT REALLY MEANS

Here's where we stand so far: ATP and CP power the first ten seconds of contraction, whereupon the anaerobic system within each working muscle takes over and provides ATP for the next 60–90 seconds. In the process, a compound called pyruvic acid is created.

If the intensity of exercise is less than maximal (just how much less is a question we'll get to later) and if it continues past the two-minute point, the aerobic system can really get down to business. The pyruvic acid is converted into a compound called *acetyl co-A*, which spins around in a process called the Krebs Cycle, throwing off ATPs left and right. The by-products of Krebs processing enter a second system called the *electron transport chain*, which squeezes out even more ATPs along with the only remains of that original glucose: water and carbon dioxide. (That's why you breathe oxygen in and carbon dioxide out, roughly speaking.) The aerobic system creates somewhere between 34 and 37 ATPs; scientists are still not sure about the exact total. Added to the two ATPs formed during anaerobic processing, one glucose molecule can yield 36 to 39 ATPs.

What happens if the intensity of exercise is at or near maximal levels during the first 90 seconds? In one word: trouble. The anaerobic system is forced to break down large amounts of glucose, and pyruvic acid is formed in great quantities. Since the aerobic system is slow to start, and works at a *very* slow pace, it can only turn a small amount of the pyruvic acid into acetyl co-A. The rest, unfortunately, is chemically transformed into *lactic acid,* or lactate. Your muscles and their enzymes can only withstand a small amount of lactate before the acid starts shutting down operations. If you work too hard, too fast, you'll feel the telltale lactic acid burn, and find that your muscles just refuse to work.

Fading in the Home Stretch

If you haven't realized it yet, you've just learned the major explanation for all those athletic successes and failures you've watched or experienced through the years. Athletes that rely on their aerobic systems, such as marathon runners, must train and compete at the speed that takes them right to their lactate-handling limit. The top coaches can actually train athletes to increase their lactate-handling ability, and to run at faster and faster speeds without going off the lactate gangplank. In fact, the best laboratory method for rating runners is not their maximum oxygen uptake, or MAX VO_2, but their V_{OBLA}, the velocity at which lactate begins to add up and seep into the bloodstream. The marathon greats run at extremely high velocities before the onset of *blood lactate accumulation* (OBLA), while we mortals start pouring out lactate at much lower speeds.

Lactate handling isn't just important to endurance athletes, however. Take a 200-meter freestyle swimmer, for example (world record of about 1 minute 48 seconds). The ATP load is being shared by the anaerobic and aerobic systems, each contributing roughly half of the total amount. If the athlete swims too fast, too early in the race, the aerobic system cannot accept all the pyruvate being formed, and lactic acid begins to accumulate. Failure in the later stages of a race is inevitably a result of lactic acid buildup from too quick an early pace or poor training.

In recent years, runners and swimmers have come to adopt a pacing method known as *negative splits* to prevent the lactate problem. Instead of starting out hard and trying to hold on, the athlete swimming negative splits swims each 50 or 100 meter leg faster than the one before. In this manner, he or she is always working within the limits of aerobic processing. As the body warms up and the aerobic juices begin to flow, the pace is gradually quickened. Many a world record has been set in this manner.

Ever wonder why all those "dream miles" on television have a no-name runner out front called a "rabbit" to set the pace? Now you know. The rabbit burns out quickly after a lap or two due to a quick pace and lactate buildup, while the elite runners behind him follow in step, preventing lactate accumulation. Many races will have two or more rabbits so that the champions end up in a true race for only the last one or two hundred meters of a 1,500. The trick is to time your last sprint so that you reach your lactate-handling capacity right at the tape. On the other hand, if you're superbly trained and have the nerve, you might try what Kip Keino tried on Jim Ryun in their Olympic 1,500 meter showdown. Banking on his ability to run at great early velocity without serious lactate buildup, Keino tore away from Ryun at the gun and never looked back. It worked.

Some of us have a genetic blessing in addition to motivation and drive. My good friend Ted Eckersdorff, a member of the doomed 1980 Olympic Modern Pentathlon Team, was found by researchers to have *twice* the normal athlete's capacity to handle lactate. He was instructed to start his sprint hundreds of meters earlier than other pentathletes since he could work at high anaerobic levels far longer than they could. If you weren't blessed like Teddy don't despair. There are several ways to increase your capacity through training. We'll get to those in Chapter 12.

At this point you should have a pretty good idea of why I've given you this physiology lesson. It would be ludicrous for anyone to think that they could design an effective fitness program *without* such knowledge. If you're an athlete, you (and your coach) should fully understand the energy requirements of your sport. Are you stressing the aerobic system? Are you stressing the anaerobic system? Are both systems working in a 60:40 ratio? Training must accurately address the physiological demands of the sport. If you're just after overall fitness, you should understand what each type of exercise can and cannot do for you. And that, finally, brings us to the big question.

IS NAUTILUS AEROBIC?

As I noted earlier, an intense Nautilus workout can easily maintain your heart rate in the 160–190 range. If you're one of the millions who have heard only half the story from those so-called "experts," you are under the impression that exercise is automatically aerobic if it raises your pulse into your target zone. (This target zone is the recommended training intensity for your age and fitness level, usually between 70% and 85% of your maximal heart rate.) Sorry, but it's just not true.

What those "experts" forgot to tell you is that heart rate is only a good indicator of aerobic intensity if the exercise involves *large* muscles, in *rhythmic* contractions, lasting at least six to eight minutes.

Does a horror movie, which can take your pulse through the roof, stimulate your aerobic system? Of course not. Does a sauna or steam bath, which drives your heart rate up in response to heat stress, require heavy aerobic help? Of course not. Heart rate can rise in response to many different stimuli, including *anaerobic* exercise. And that's where Nautilus enters the picture.

Here's why Nautilus is only 45%–60% aerobic: each machine trains one specific muscle or muscle group. The first ten seconds of the exercise are fueled by ATP and CP. The next 60–90 seconds are largely anaerobic. Toward the end of this interval the aerobic system comes to bear about half the load. You're working at high intensity, and both nervous system reflexes and the need for more blood cause your heart rate to climb. Then, boom, you've completed your twelve repetitions, and you're off to the next machine. And a *different, fresh* muscle. First ten seconds: ATP and CP. Next 60–90 seconds: mostly anaerobic, partly aerobic. Since each muscle is worked for only 12–15 repetitions, or about 90 seconds, the muscle's aerobic system is never given a chance to get fully cranked up. Just as it begins to supply ATP, you're off to a new muscle and a new aerobic system.

What does it all mean? You're going to see a lot of changes in your body from Nautilus, but aerobic benefits won't likely be among them. Most importantly to those of you interested in burning off some excess fat: Nautilus won't do it. A good, hard, 20-minute workout will burn 150 to 200 calories, but the duration won't be great enough to cause your body to start breaking down the fat stores. What's more, the calories will come mainly from glucose or its storage form, glycogen. The task of burning fat will be left to lower intensity, longer duration aerobic exercise. You'll get the full story on *that* in Chapter 11.

3
YOUR OPERATING MANUAL: MUSCLES

Philosophers down through the ages have commented on man's preoccupation with muscle. Among the treasures we live by are these favorites:

"A muscle in the hand is worth two in the bush."

"A journey of a thousand miles begins with the first muscle."

"Monkey see, muscle do."

"Speak softly and carry a big muscle."

Et cetera.

Seriously, it's time to get down to the business that brought you here in the first place: muscle.

First up is an explanation of the structure and types of muscle. We'll start with the overall view then work our way down to the tiny proteins which do the work of contraction. If you thought muscle was just muscle, think again: we humans possess *four* distinct types of skeletal muscle (the kind that moves your bones and your body).

As my anatomy professors always said, "function follows structure." After learning how muscle is put together we'll see how it works. This time we'll start small then work

our way up to the various types of contractions (isokinetics, eccentrics, etc.).

Finally, we'll tie everything together and lay out the implications of all this for Nautilus training in the section on motor control—how the brain runs the show.

STRUCTURE

The Three Classes of Muscle

You've already heard about skeletal muscles. They're the ones that you're here to read about. They generally run from one bone to another across a joint, and, by contracting, create movement. You'll find two other classes of muscle in your body, though. Cardiac muscle contracts somewhat like skeletal muscle, but has several microscopic differences. Most interesting of these is its "on-board electronic ignition." Certain cardiac muscle cells are actually tiny electrical generators, and the signals they send out tell the entire heart when to contract. These structures are called "pacemaker cells," and obviously gave rise to the idea for external

9

devices that heart disease patients can wear.

The third general class of muscle is called smooth or visceral. It also is microscopically different from skeletal muscle, and is found in the walls of your body's internal gut organs (the "viscera"). The stomach is probably the best example of smooth muscle.

A Word on Contraction

Before I continue on I should remind you of the fact that muscle can only be asked to shorten or contract. The proteins that actually do the work *cannot* push outward. How then can we accomplish a pushing movement?

Through the pairing of muscles on opposite sides of a bone or limb, that's how. Take a quick look around your body and note how muscles all appear in pairs. Take your arm as an example. Hold it straight out in front of you with the palm facing up. When the biceps on the top surface of the upper arm contracts, it brings the hand and forearm closer to the shoulder. The triceps, located on the bottom surface of the upper arm, also attaches to the forearm. It is being stretched when the biceps does its thing. Want to push with the hand and forearm? All the triceps needs do is contract and pull the forearm back to starting position. Voila! Pushing movement through contraction of a muscle.

The Overall Picture

Skeletal muscles with common names like the hamstrings and quadriceps may actually be composed of anywhere from two to four muscles. Other muscles may arise from one bone in two or three different parts, then join to insert on (attach to) a second bone as one. (Nothing's ever simple, is it?) Here are the more important examples of confusing names:

- Quadriceps: four muscles on the front of the thigh. Their names: *vastus lateralis, vastus medialis, vastus intermedius,* and *rectus femoris.*
- Hamstrings: three muscles behind the thigh. Their names: *semitendinosus, semi-*

membranosus, and *biceps femoris.*
- Triceps: three different "heads" or origins from the shoulder, one attachment to the forearm. Different exercises must be used to fully develop all three heads.
- Biceps: two different heads from the scapula, one attachment to the forearm.
- Deltoids: the three shoulder muscles. Their names: *anterior* (front) *deltoid, middle deltoid, posterior* (rear) *deltoid.* Different exercises are needed to best develop all three.

Fibers, Fibrils, and Filaments

Now that we've straightened out that terminology, we can get down to the business of muscle fibers. The analogy that best explains the fine structure of muscle is a phone company cable. The cable as a whole is really little more than a bundle that packages the many smaller cables which transmit the phone calls.

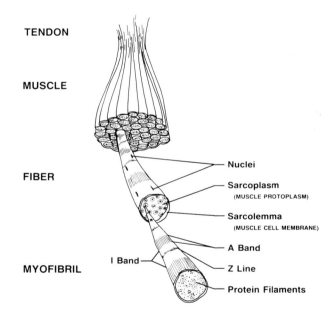

Muscle can be pictured as a large phone company cable containing many smaller cables. From *The Physiological Basis of Physical Education and Sport* by D. Mathews and E. L. Fox. © 1981 Saunders. Reprinted by permission of Holt, Rinehart and Winston, CBS College Publishing.

A muscle fiber is, in the same way, little more than a bundle of smaller fibers called *myofibrils.* These structures in turn contain the protein strands which do the actual contracting, the *myofilaments*. One muscle fiber may contain scores of myofibrils, and each myofibril contains scores of myofilaments. It has been estimated that there are more than a quarter of a billion muscle fibers in the average man!

FUNCTION

The Contractile Proteins

There are four types of protein in muscle. The two largest, known as *actin* and *myosin*, are called *contractile proteins* because they actually link up and shorten to create muscular force. The two smaller proteins, *troponin* and *tropomyosin*, are part of the on-off switch mechanism for actin and myosin.

Contrary to what all those powdered-protein pushers would have you believe, only 22% of muscle is protein. In fact, more than 70% of muscle is good old water. There is not a shred of evidence that any athlete needs supplemental protein if he/she pays even the slightest attention to good nutrition. We'll have more on that later.

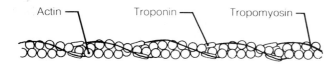

Thin Filament

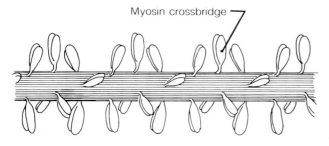

Thick Filament

Troponin and tropomyosin proteins encircle the thin strands of actin protein. Crossbridges extend from the thick myosin protein toward actin. Reprinted by permission of Saunders College Publishing and W. H. Freeman and Co./Scientific American.

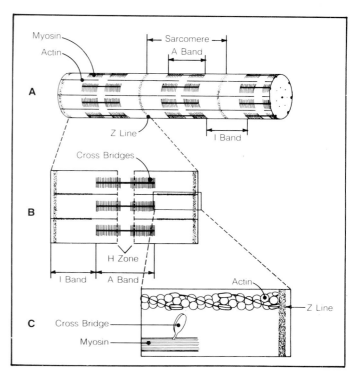

A myofibril (A) is made up of thousands of "sarcomeres" in series. A sarcomere (B) is the unit of contraction, and lies between two Z-lines. Shown in closeup (C) is the crossbridge that extends from thick myosin to thin actin. From *Sports Physiology* by E. L. Fox. © 1979 Saunders. Reprinted by permission of Holt, Rinehart and Winston, CBS College Publishing.

The Contraction Process

Muscle contraction begins with a signal from the nervous system. When the electrical impulse arrives at the muscle it is rapidly transmitted up and down the length and depth of the muscle through a system of *tubules*. When the message reaches each of the thousands of on-off sites or *receptors*, a little package of calcium is released. Mom was right when she nagged you to drink your milk!

The calcium exerts an inhibiting effect on the intertwined troponin-tropomyosin proteins, which to this point have been keeping actin and myosin apart. When their effect is briefly removed by the calcium, the actin and myosin proteins can go about the business of contracting.

To best understand the process of contraction we need to look at one, single functional unit of actin and myosin, called a *sarcomere*. At each end of the sarcomere is a thick anchoring structure called a *Z-disc*. Extending into the sarcomere from each Z-disc are thin strands of actin protein, which just barely overlap the thick strands of myosin found in the middle of the sarcomere. Each of these myosin strands has little hooklike structures which extend out toward the actin. They are known as *cross-bridges*.

When the calcium is released by the nerve cells, and the effect of troponin and tropomyosin is removed, a strange thing happens to the actin and myosin. For reasons still not fully understood, the following automatic process occurs:

- The proteins undergo a *conformational* (shape) change.
- The cross-bridges attach to the actin protein strands.
- The cross-bridges *rotate* and *pull* microscopically inward on the actin filaments and Z-discs.
- The sarcomere shortens since both Z-discs have been drawn inward.

When many sarcomeres shorten at once, the muscle fiber and then the muscle contract.

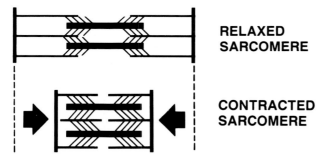

RELAXED SARCOMERE

CONTRACTED SARCOMERE

When the crossbridges attach to the actin proteins and pull, the sarcomere (and muscle as a whole) shortens. Note that the thick myosin protein does not itself shorten, but rather the Z-lines are pulled inward.

It is *not* the energy from ATP breakdown that allows this to occur, though most textbooks will tell you that. The process of contraction occurs automatically when calcium inhibits troponin and tropomyosin. ATP *is*

needed, however, to allow the cross-bridges to release and return to their ready position for the next pull. When you flexed and extended your forearm in our earlier example you were seeing the results of thousands of pulls and releases by the cross-bridges; the pulls dependent on calcium, the releases fueled by the energy from ATP breakdown.

We've now gone as deep as we can go in understanding how muscle works. The ATP created through the anaerobic and aerobic systems is needed to allow actin and myosin to work smoothly in the contraction/relaxation process. Exceed your ATP production capability and there's just no way to go on!

The Four Fiber Types

Getting more specific, there are actually several different types of actin and myosin. The speed with which a muscle can contract is heavily dependent on the kind of myosin contained within the muscle. *Heavy meromyosin,* or HMM, is capable of rapid ATP breakdown and is found in fast muscles. *Light meromyosin,* or LMM, is characteristic of slower muscles.

What we actually find on analysis of human muscle is that four different categories appear. Several years back the terms *fast-twitch* and *slow-twitch* were used to describe muscles, but we've learned since that there are *three* types of fast-twitch muscle.

As seen in the table on page 13, scientists have chosen to create four naming systems for the various types of skeletal muscle rather than making it easy for us.

Slow muscle (type-S), which turns out to be slow only in comparison to the fast fibers, is the endurance fiber used by distance athletes. It is your most aerobically powerful fiber, with a heavy-duty supply of aerobic enzymes, blood vessels, and an oxygen-holding endurance compound called *myoglobin.* It can create little force, but it's capable of contracting for long periods of time without fatigue. The leg muscles of elite marathon runners are quite often composed almost entirely of slow muscle fibers.

Fast muscle fibers differ in endurance capa-

GETTING TO KNOW YOUR FIBER TYPES

Characteristic	Type I/SO/S	Type IIa/FO/FR	Type IIab/FOG/FI	Type IIb/FG/FF
Color	Red	Pink	Pink	White
Speed of contraction	Slow	Fast	Fast	Fast
Fatigability	Highly resistant	Moderately resistant	Lower resistance	Highly fatigable
Aerobic capacity	Highest	Moderate	Lower	Lowest
Anaerobic capacity	Lowest	High	High	Highest
Capillaries per fiber	Many	Few	Few	Fewest
Size of fibers	Smallest	Large	Large	Largest
Contribution to total force output of muscle	less than 5%	10%	10%	75%

bilities more than in speed. The *fast-oxidative* (FO) fibers have fairly good endurance. The term *oxidative*, by the way, refers to the aerobic machinery within the FO fibers. The *fast-glycolytic* (FG) fibers are very fast, very powerful, but have no endurance. The word *glycolytic* refers to the anaerobic machinery in these fibers. The deltoids and triceps of elite shotputters, for example, are often almost entirely FG fibers. Intermediate in speed, power, and endurance are the *fast-oxidative-glycolytic* (FOG) fibers, with both aerobic and anaerobic machinery within.

It's All Genetic

Unfortunately for those of us with dreams of athletic greatness, our fiber type percentages appear to be genetically determined. Most of us are born with a relatively even mix of fast and slow fibers, which to a great extent prevents us from being major successes in any sport we try. The greats in sprinting and the power events are almost always blessed with high FG fiber percentages, and most of our marathon greats have lower bodies just loaded with type-S fibers.

There *is* some good news, however: scores

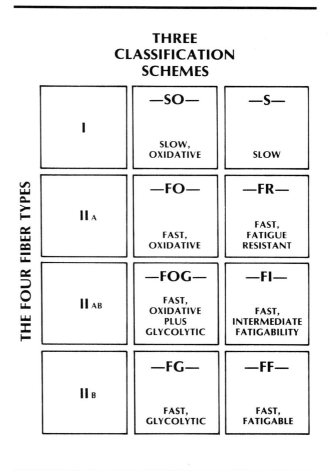

THREE CLASSIFICATION SCHEMES

THE FOUR FIBER TYPES

I	—SO— SLOW, OXIDATIVE	—S— SLOW
II A	—FO— FAST, OXIDATIVE	—FR— FAST, FATIGUE RESISTANT
II AB	—FOG— FAST, OXIDATIVE PLUS GLYCOLYTIC	—FI— FAST, INTERMEDIATE FATIGABILITY
II B	—FG— FAST, GLYCOLYTIC	—FF— FAST, FATIGABLE

of factors contribute to athletic success, and it's not terribly unusual to see a sub 2:20 marathoner with only a moderate percentage of slow fibers in his legs. As I noted in the last chapter, several elite marathoners make up for less-than-spectacular maximum oxygen consumption (Max VO$_2$) numbers by having inhumanly high V$_{OBLA}$ numbers (high velocities before the onset of blood lactate accumulation).

Whether you are genetically blessed or not, the only truly important challenge you face is exceeding the goals you set for yourself. And that's as true of housewives and executives as it is of Olympic athletes.

The Strength Curve

Things would be a lot simpler if muscles all ran in a perfectly straight line from one bone to the next. They don't. Or if they were all simple arrangements of side-by-side fibers. They're not. Actually, muscles run around, through, and over bones (well, almost) before they attach, and are found with several different internal structures. The result of all this confusion is the *strength curve*.

When we measure the strength of a muscle, or the amount of force that it can create, we see that the number changes as we move the limb through its *range of motion*. Someone who can create 100 pounds of force in a biceps curl with his upper and lower arms held at a 90° angle might only be able to create 70 pounds at 135° and 30 pounds at 170°. If you plot the strength at five or more points from start to finish, you'd have yourself a strength curve.

Because each muscle attaches to its target bone in a unique way, and because there are several different internal formations that muscle can take, every muscle has its own, unique strength curve. Some, like that of the quadriceps, look like an inverted and flattened letter "U." Others, like the hamstrings strength curve, show a brief rise in force output then a rapid decrease through the rest of the range of motion.

All well and good, you say. But what does this have to do with strength training? Here comes the physics lesson: the work load that

a barbell or weight stack places on your muscles is *not* measured solely by what it weighs. The physicist measures something more meaningful called *torque*, or turning force, which the load is applying to the limbs. Place your arm in that 90° biceps curl position again. Now imagine that a weight is trying to turn or torque your lower arm downward at the elbow joint. The *amount* of torque is determined by *two* things: how much the load weighs and how far the load is from the joint.

To figure out the true or *effective resistance* of a barbell, draw vertical lines downward from the barbell and the center of the rotating joint, then connect the two lines with a third, perpendicular line (see the drawing that follows). To get torque or effective resistance, multiply the weight of the load by the perpendicular distance, or *moment arm*. This figure will be labeled as *inch-pounds* if you measure in those units.

THE BICEPS CURL:
EFFECTIVE RESISTANCE WITH A 30 POUND BARBELL

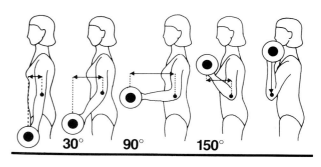

2 inches 30 lbs.	6 inches 30 lbs.	10 inches 30 lbs.	6 inches 30 lbs.	0 inches 30 lbs.
60 in. lbs.	180 in. lbs.	300 in. lbs.	180 in. lbs.	0 in. lbs.

The "effective resistance" of a 30-pound barbell changes according to the law of physics. The load your muscles feel is obtained by multiplying the barbell weight by the "moment arm," or the horizontal arrows.

Watch how much the effective resistance of a barbell or weight load changes during a curl: a moment arm of two inches on a 30-pound barbell yields a torque of 60 inch-pounds, while a 10-inch moment arm on the same barbell gives a torque of 300 inch-pounds, a *fivefold* increase!

Here's what we have so far: Each muscle has its own, unique strength curve due to anatomical differences, and at the same time, a barbell exercise has *its* own variations due to physics and gravity. There is therefore a fundamental mismatch between muscle and barbell. The muscle may exhibit increasing strength as it moves through the range of motion, while the barbell load may be getting progressively easier. Or, of course, the opposite could happen. What we need is an intelligent barbell, one that gets heavier when the muscle increases in its force output capacity, and decreases when the muscle gets weaker.

Son of a gun—that's what a Nautilus machine does!

The Types of Contractions

And you thought a contraction was just a contraction. Unfortunately, it's not that simple!

If a muscle tries to shorten or contract, and it does, you have a *concentric* contraction. If it tries to shorten and finds that it can't, and therefore does not change in length, you have an *isometric* contraction. If an external force pulls a muscle out (lengthens it) while it continues to attempt to shorten, you have an *eccentric* contraction. Think of fighting to lower a weight with the same muscle that lifted it as an eccentric contraction.

The first three definitions were easy. It's the next two that are tough. According to the old definition, an *isotonic* contraction is one where the load remains constant through the entire movement. A 50-pound barbell curl would therefore be isotonic, right? Wrong. As we just explained above, the laws of physics change the *resultant load* of the barbell as you curl it. While it will always weigh 50 pounds on a scale, the muscles curling the weight see a load that increases more than *twelvefold* between the starting and 90° positions.

The last category of contraction is *isokinetic*. Strictly speaking, isokinetic means same movement, which seems pretty dumb. The term is commonly used to describe contractions that are made at a constant velocity. It turns out that there are only three devices that allow you to train at true constant velocities, and the cheapest of them costs $28,000.

What purpose does isokinetics serve?

One major problem with barbells and Nautilus or Nautilus-type machines is that of momentum or intertia. Once you start the weight moving, whether it's on a bar or in a weight stack, it has its own momentum. If you exert too great a force too quickly, the weight may actually pick up enough momentum to move *on its own*. Of course, once the weight is on its own, the muscles are doing no work and cannot be trained. This problem limits you in the speeds and forces at which you can train.

True isokinetic devices have the ability to soak up whatever forces you create and keep you at whatever speed you select. Dial in 60 degrees of rotation per second then work away. No matter how much force your muscles may create, you will move at a speed no greater than 60° per second. Top speed on present devices is only 300° per second, however, which is not terribly high when compared to some athletic movements.

Shall we dump Nautilus, then, and head for an isokinetic training device? Hold your horses. First of all, there's no solid proof that isokinetic training has any greater effect on athletic performance or strength gains than good Nautilus training. Second, feedback to the user on most isokinetic-type devices is generally poor. It is difficult to watch a little pointer on a little dial and know exactly what you accomplished in that last set. Finally, the major strength of isokinetics turns out to be its major weakness. If for any reason your muscle has imbalances in the strength curve (unusually weak points), an isokinetic device will see that weakness and return it. Give it 300 pounds and it'll give you 300 back. Give it 20, though, and you'll get 20 back.

For the millions of people with abnormal strength curves, isokinetic devices will *perpetuate* their problems. Are you weak in the middle of a movement? At the ends? Your force output will drop, and the isokinetic device will kindly show you less force.

This is where the Nautilus cam shines. Each cam is designed for the ideal strength curve of the muscle(s) being trained. As we'll learn later in the section on variable resistance, the cam actually *changes* the load as you move through the exercise. Continued training on cam-based Nautilus machines can actually correct imbalances in your strength curve.

Though Mike Fulton, M.D., orthopedic surgeon and Clinic Director at Nautilus headquarters, has detailed this process in scores of patients, I thought you'd like to hear about the changes in my own quadriceps over one summer of Nautilus training. I began the summer with marked weakness at both full flexion and full extension of the lower leg. Through nine weeks of training, both ends of the curve had been brought up gradually, so that I became stronger.

Now that I've settled all that, where does Nautilus fit in? It's not isokinetic. It's not isotonic or isometric. What is it? Unfortunately, there isn't a scientific term to describe it. Let's just call it *variable resistance exercise*.

GETTING BIGGER AND STRONGER

What happens if you learn your lessons well and strength train with good form, on good equipment, with high intensity? The very first thing is purely neurological. Before your muscles change at all, your brain becomes more efficient at using what it's got.

The change you've been waiting for is called *hypertrophy*, an increase in the size of the muscle. Four changes explain hypertrophy:

- an increase in the number of myofibrils
- an increase in the amount of actin and myosin proteins
- an increase in the number of blood vessels within the muscle
- an increase in the amount and strength of the tendon tissue running through the muscle

Since women tend to have about 30 times

less *testosterone* than men (the male sex hormone that enables hypertrophy), they also tend to show less hypertrophy. They *do* show equal percentage strength gains, though, which can be explained by greater neurological efficiency and a phenomenon known as *contractile element packing*. This

CONTRACTILE ELEMENT PACKING

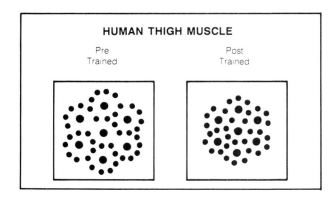

One likely explanation for an increase in strength without an increase in size (women, pay attention!) is a denser packing of existing muscle fibers.

25-cent phrase simply means that more actin and myosin proteins can be packed into the same amount of space as before, increasing strength without increasing size.

The final change which muscle may undergo is *hyperplasia*, an increase in the number of muscle fibers. Though this is still a hotly debated question, it appears that muscle fibers may split in two after growing to a particular size. The two smaller fibers may then grow to that same size and split again. This is a technical question that really doesn't affect us, so let's just move on . . .

The big question, of course, is how does one cause hypertrophy? Well, we're not ready for that answer yet. It'll have to wait just a *few* more pages . . .

ANTERIOR VIEW OF THE MUSCULAR SYSTEM

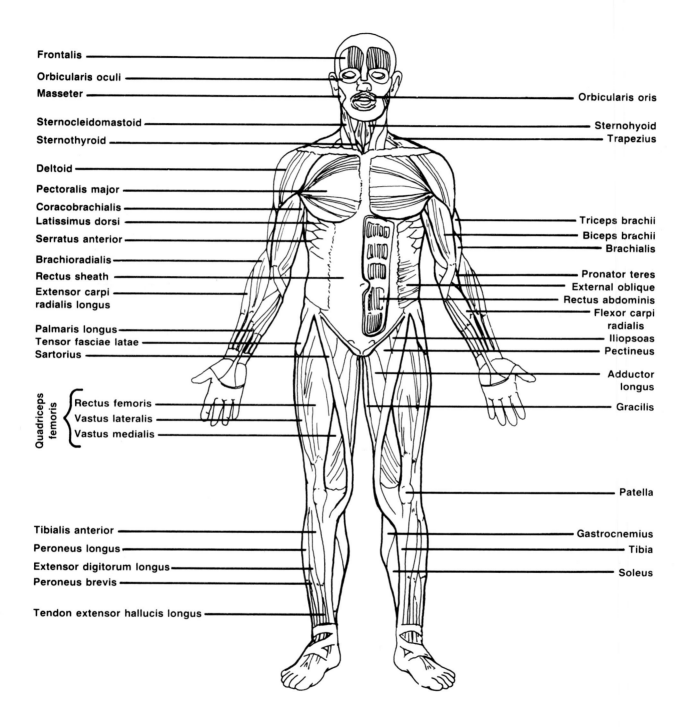

Frontalis

Orbicularis oculi

Masseter

Orbicularis oris

Sternocleidomastoid

Sternhyoid

Sternothyroid

Trapezius

Deltoid

Pectoralis major

Coracobrachialis

Latissimus dorsi

Triceps brachii

Serratus anterior

Biceps brachii

Brachialis

Brachioradialis

Rectus sheath

Pronator teres

Extensor carpi
radialis longus

External oblique

Rectus abdominis

Flexor carpi
radialis

Palmaris longus

Tensor fasciae latae

Iliopsoas

Sartorius

Pectineus

Adductor
longus

Quadriceps femoris
{ Rectus femoris
Vastus lateralis
Vastus medialis

Gracilis

Patella

Tibialis anterior

Gastrocnemius

Peroneus longus

Tibia

Extensor digitorum longus

Soleus

Peroneus brevis

Tendon extensor hallucis longus

POSTERIOR VIEW OF THE MUSCULAR SYSTEM

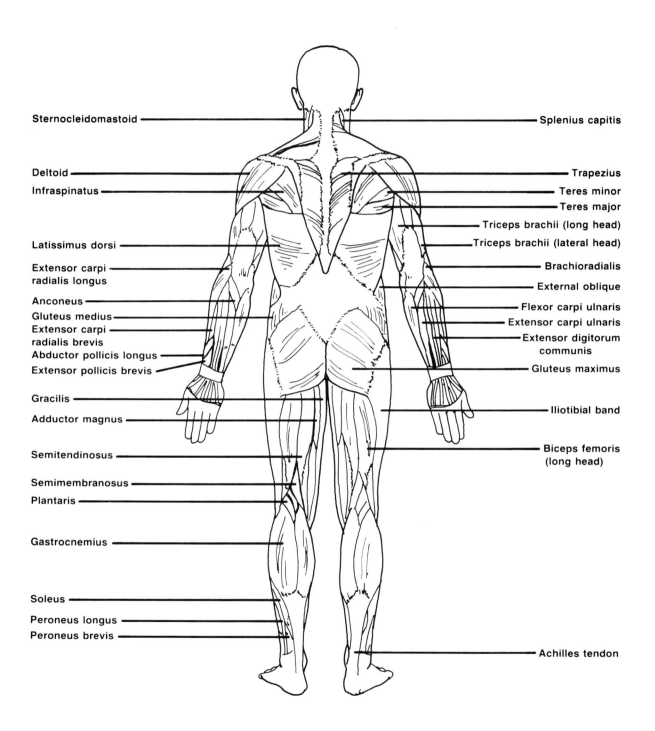

Sternocleidomastoid

Deltoid
Infraspinatus

Latissimus dorsi

Extensor carpi
radialis longus

Anconeus
Gluteus medius
Extensor carpi
radialis brevis
Abductor pollicis longus
Extensor pollicis brevis

Gracilis
Adductor magnus

Semitendinosus

Semimembranosus
Plantaris

Gastrocnemius

Soleus
Peroneus longus
Peroneus brevis

Splenius capitis

Trapezius
Teres minor
Teres major
Triceps brachii (long head)
Triceps brachii (lateral head)
Brachioradialis
External oblique
Flexor carpi ulnaris
Extensor carpi ulnaris
Extensor digitorum
communis
Gluteus maximus

Iliotibial band

Biceps femoris
(long head)

Achilles tendon

MUSCULAR SYSTEM OF THE LOWER LIMBS

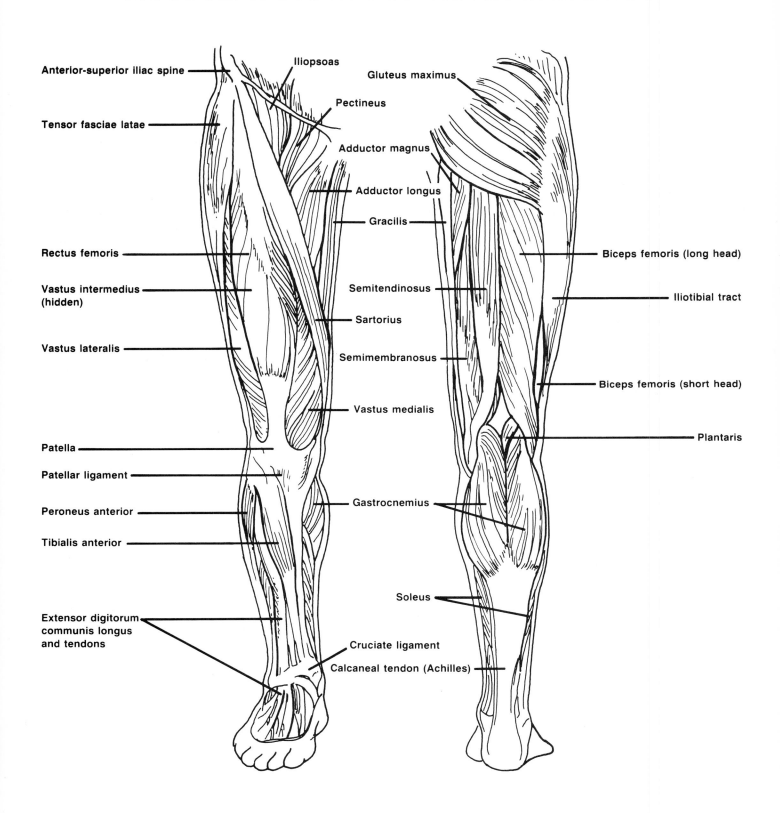

Anterior-superior iliac spine

Iliopsoas

Gluteus maximus

Pectineus

Tensor fasciae latae

Adductor magnus

Adductor longus

Gracilis

Rectus femoris

Biceps femoris (long head)

Vastus intermedius (hidden)

Semitendinosus

Iliotibial tract

Sartorius

Vastus lateralis

Semimembranosus

Biceps femoris (short head)

Vastus medialis

Plantaris

Patella

Patellar ligament

Peroneus anterior

Gastrocnemius

Tibialis anterior

Extensor digitorum communis longus and tendons

Soleus

Cruciate ligament

Calcaneal tendon (Achilles)

ANTERIOR SURFACE OF THE ARM

POSTERIOR SURFACE OF THE ARM

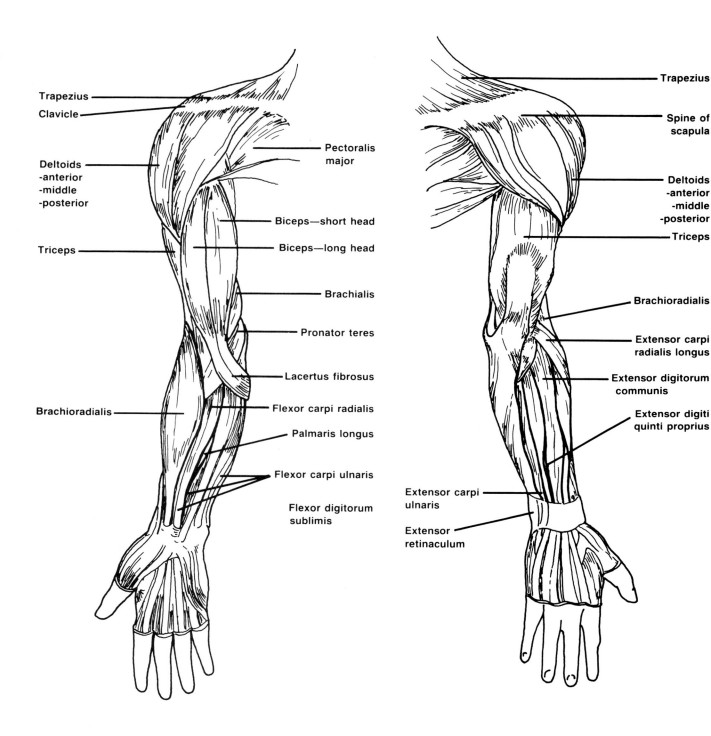

Trapezius

Clavicle

Deltoids
-anterior
-middle
-posterior

Triceps

Brachioradialis

Pectoralis major

Biceps—short head

Biceps—long head

Brachialis

Pronator teres

Lacertus fibrosus

Flexor carpi radialis

Palmaris longus

Flexor carpi ulnaris

Flexor digitorum sublimis

Trapezius

Spine of scapula

Deltoids
-anterior
-middle
-posterior

Triceps

Brachioradialis

Extensor carpi radialis longus

Extensor digitorum communis

Extensor digiti quinti proprius

Extensor carpi ulnaris

Extensor retinaculum

ANTERIOR VIEW OF THE TRUNK

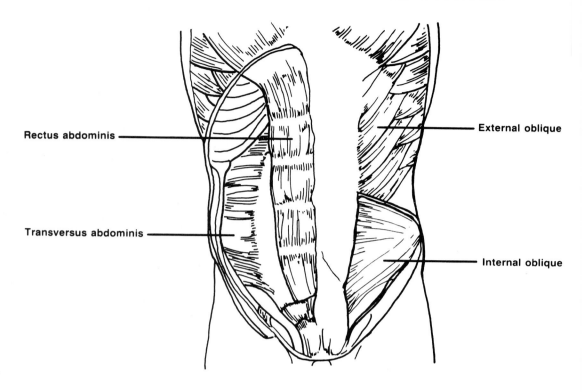

Rectus abdominis

Transversus abdominis

External oblique

Internal oblique

POSTERIOR VIEW OF THE TRUNK

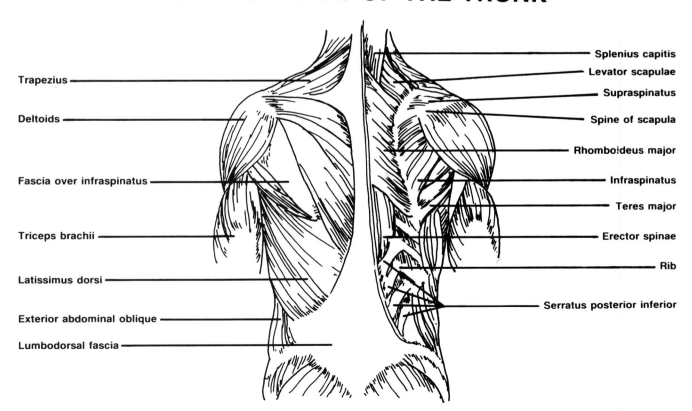

Trapezius

Deltoids

Fascia over infraspinatus

Triceps brachii

Latissimus dorsi

Exterior abdominal oblique

Lumbodorsal fascia

Splenius capitis

Levator scapulae

Supraspinatus

Spine of scapula

Rhomboideus major

Infraspinatus

Teres major

Erector spinae

Rib

Serratus posterior inferior

CONTROL

Report at 0700 Hours

Now that I've got you in a military mood, I can tell you in one word how the brain controls muscle: *recruitment.* Just as Uncle Sam calls up soldiers when he needs them, the brain recruits muscle fibers through its motor nerves. Furthermore, the brain follows a relatively fixed order in recruiting muscle, much as the government followed the numbers drawn in the draft lottery.

The system is actually pretty ingenious, involving the amount of electrical current necessary to turn the muscle fibers on. The slow or type-S fibers are the easiest to turn on, requiring only a slight current. It requires a bit more juice to turn on the FO fibers, and still more for the FOGs. Most difficult to excite electrically are the FG fibers.

Now, the brain is lazy, the ultraconservative organ; it *never* does more than it has to in accomplishing a task. Let's go back to our barbell curl example. The brain will try to accomplish the curl with the type-S fibers. If these can't create enough force, more juice will be sent to the muscle to recruit the FO and FOG fibers. If even these fail, the brain will have to turn up the current one last time for the FG fibers. This process is described as *orderly recruitment,* for the brain does not run about haphazardly choosing muscle fibers to turn on.

If you were paying attention in the last paragraph, you may have realized that I talked only about force; velocity was not mentioned. Very simply, the brain is far more concerned about the force it must generate than the velocity. It does not say, "Gee, this guy wants to move fast. I better turn on fast fibers." It cannot *preferentially recruit* fast fi-

bers. The brain *does* ask, "How much force must be created to move this load (barbell, baseball bat, whatever) at the desired velocity?" It then tries to send a message of sufficient electrical intensity to turn on the necessary fibers. If enough current arrives to turn on the FG fibers, we automatically know that the S, FO, and FOG fibers are also on.

This knowledge is *absolutely critical* to how you train. Many coaches and poorly-informed salespeople will have you believe that speed on the track or in the pool can only be created by fast, explosive strength training. This completely disregards the principles of motor control. If you try to work at very high speeds in the weightroom, you'll be forced to use light weights. (Obviously, the heavier the weight the slower it can be moved.) Do that and the brain says, "It won't take much *force* to move 30 pounds at that high velocity. I'll send down just enough current for the S and FO fibers." The end result is that you don't recruit the fibers most important to high-speed movement on the field or in the pool, the FGs. Give yourself a heavy load in the weightroom and you force the brain to recruit the full complement of muscle fibers.

That, then, is what hypertrophy is all about. The fibers that respond most quickly to strength training, and grow the largest, are the FGs. They can only be recruited if the brain is asked to move a heavy load. High-speed training is dangerous and less productive than slow, high-intensity work.

For maximal athletic success, slow but brutal Nautilus training must be combined with high-speed *skill* training. The only way to run or swim fast in competition is to run or swim fast in training, but the process is definitely aided by good strength work. You'll get the lowdown on combining Nautilus, skill, and aerobic training in Chapter 11.

4

YOUR OPERATING MANUAL: FEEDING THE MACHINE

From an efficiency standpoint, it's too bad that fueling your own engine is so much harder than fueling your car's engine. The only decision you face at the filling station is the octane rating of the gasoline, while good nutrition requires selections that intelligently incorporate the six classes of nutrients: carbohydrates, fats, proteins, water, vitamins, and minerals.

Other than the need to stuff your face, these nutrients fulfill seven major roles in bodily functions:

- maintenance and repair of body tissues
- growth of new muscle, bone, and organ tissue
- regulation of the chemical processes that occur in the body
- energy for muscle contraction
- nerve conduction
- gland secretion
- reproduction

While good nutrition requires some work, it's *not* as bad as all those health food store owners would have you believe. This chapter will be your guide to distinguishing fact from fiction in nutrition, and will help improve the quality of daily life as well as athletic performance.

Our battle plan: first up is a discussion of the six nutrients. We'll then move to metabolism and the lowdown on weight control, body composition, eating schedules, and meal timing. Closing the chapter will be advice to take to the supermarket and kitchen: how to select, prepare, and eat.

THE NUTRIENTS

Carbohydrates

Far from being villains and the sure cause of obesity, carbohydrates are actually critical to bodily function and are needed in large quantities. The minimum percentage of your daily caloric intake that should come from carbos is 60%, and many nutritionists recommend 70% and up if you're physically active!

Carbohydrates, whether in their "simple"

form (like table sugar), or complex form (potatoes), must be broken down to glucose before the body can make use of them. Glucose is then transported throughout the body via the blood, where it can suffer several fates:

- it may be used immediately by the body's cells for energy
- it may be stored in the muscle or liver in long chains called "glycogen"
- it may be metabolically converted into fat for long-term storage if glycogen stores have reached their peak
- it may continue to circulate in the blood, being drawn upon by muscles or other cells for energy whenever needed

At least 75% of your daily carbohydrate calories should come from the complex forms: hot cereals, pasta, fresh fruits and vegetables, beans (except soybeans), whole grains (rice, barley, corn, etc.), and whole-grain breads. There is room for simple carbohydrate calories (like fruit juices, dried or canned fruit, cake, candy, soft drinks, honey), but they are frequently poor in other nutrients and provide little fiber (which aids digestion).

A technique known as "carbohydrate loading" has gotten a great deal of publicity lately. By first emptying your body of all its stored glycogen, then reloading carbos in superhuman amounts, the muscles very often store far more glycogen than is normally possible.

Why would one want to do this? Endurance athletes run on both glycogen and fat. Even the leanest athlete has enough fat calories for an ultramarathon: at 9 calories per gram, and 454 grams per pound, each pound of fat in your body yields 4,100 calories of energy. At a caloric cost of 100 per mile, one pound of fat could power you for 40 miles. Glucose, however, only provides 4 calories of energy per gram, and is stored (as glycogen) in far smaller amounts. It is to the athlete's advantage to have plenty of easily-utilized glycogen right in the muscle. Carbo loading promises to give you more muscle glycogen than a normal diet would.

The two problems with carbo loading are that (a) it doesn't work for everyone and (b) the process of depleting glycogen first is

quite unpleasant. Starting about six days before competition, you are faced with two to three days of almost zero-carbohydrate diet. This wipes you out both physically and mentally. When you enter the stuff-your-face phase, you find yourself bloating like a blimp: every gram of glycogen you add is stored with 2.7 grams of water. Add one pound of glycogen and you'll add three pounds of water!

My advice: Skip it. The technique is too painful and doesn't work for enough people to make it worthwhile.

Fats

Though we think of fat solely as the stuff that ruins the way we look each summer, there are really three kinds within the body, and each plays an important role.

The most visible form of fat is *triglycerides*. This is the type of fat you store for energy, and each molecule is composed of one *glycerol* cluster and one *fatty acid* cluster. These latter compounds are the ones that can be either *saturated* or *unsaturated,* and unless you've been off vacationing in Siberia for the past ten years, you are aware that saturated fats have been linked to heart disease. Fats that are solid at room temperature or are found in meats and dairy products are usually saturated, while most commercially available cooking oils are polyunsaturated.

The second type of fat in the body is called *cholesterol.* Like carbohydrates, cholesterol has achieved villainous status without great justification. There is, to this date, no terribly strong evidence linking cholesterol in the diet to heart disease. It *does* make sense from a safety standpoint to cut back on saturated fat and cholesterol intake, but don't lose any sleep over an extra omelette. Cholesterol is important for the production of hormones, and the body can actually produce one to two grams a day of cholesterol even if you eliminate it completely from your diet.

Phospholipids are the third type of fat, and are found in the walls of all your body's cells. They are composed of phosphorous and lipid (fat).

As noted in Chapter 2, it takes at least 30 minutes of aerobic exercise for the body to start breaking down fat for energy. As exercise continues, fat gradually becomes the *major* source of fuel for muscle. Since fat is stored in so much greater amounts than glycogen, an endurance athlete would want to maximize his fat usage and save his glycogen for late-in-the-race sprinting. This role of fat in saving glycogen for the later stages of exercise is called *glycogen sparing*. It turns out that endurance training improves the body's ability to use fat during exercise. One major study showed that rats who had trained on a treadmill were 3.3 times more efficient fat burners than non-runners. Planning on doing any long-distance running or swimming? Make sure you get plenty of long-distance work done during training. Among other things it will train you to be a better fat burner.

While the average American consumes about 40% of his/her daily calories from fat, scientists and nutritionists suggest that this be reduced to about 20%. While fat *is* necessary for several bodily functions, it is calorie dense (nine calories per gram versus four for carbos and proteins) and has been tentatively linked to cancer and heart disease. A small amount of fat will satisfy your metabolic needs and retard feelings of hunger, but be careful beyond that.

Protein

Muscle tissue, structural integrity, enzymes, genetic material, hemoglobin, hormones—all these are uses of protein in the body. You probably need to eat *at least* two mountain lions a day to get that much protein into your body! Wrong.

You're probably a victim of years of false and misleading advertising by protein salesmen. The body needs protein—nine *amino acids* it can't produce, prefixed *essential*, and eleven it can produce, tabbed *nonessential*—in almost unbelievably small amounts. The recommended intake of protein for healthy adults is 0.9 grams per kilogram of body weight; for example, 63 grams a day for a 154-pound male. The recommendation increases to 1.5 grams per kilogram for extremely active adults, bringing the total daily intake to 105 grams for the 154-pounder.

What kinds of food need you eat to obtain 105 grams of protein? Two chicken breasts, a two-ounce piece of cod, and miscellaneous milk, nuts, veggies, etc. Or, in other words, a normal, three-meal day, easily at or under your caloric needs but satisfying all your protein needs. *No protein supplement in that list!* That wonder pill you've heard about—Spirulina protein? Works out to about $75 a *pound*, and *is not* a particularly good source of the nine essential amino acids. *Complete proteins*, containing all nine essentials, are found in poultry, fish, meats (keep 'em lean), milk, and eggs. You can and should eat grains and legumes, but stick to the major sources listed above for security. Use the sidebar on page 26 and Appendix II as your selection guide.

PROTEINS

Most proteins are composed of twenty-two constituents called *amino acids*. Those that can be produced in the body are called *nonessential*. This does not mean that they are unnecessary, just that they need not be consumed in the diet. The nine amino acids that cannot be produced by the body, and must therefore be ingested, are called *essential* amino acids.

Essential Amino Acids		*Nonessential Amino Acids*	
Histidine	Phenylalanine	Alanine	Hydroxyglutamic Acid
Isoleucine	Threonine	Arginine	Hydroxproline
Leucine	Tryptophan	Aspartic Acid	Proline
Lysine	Valine	Citrulline	Serine
Methionine		Norleucine	Tyrosine
		Glutamic Acid	Cystine
		Glycine	

PROTEIN VALUES OF SOME COMMON FOODS

Food	Measure	Protein (gm)
Chicken, breast	2.7 oz.	25.0
Tuna fish	3 oz.	24.0
Beef, round	3 oz.	24.0
Lamb, leg	3 oz.	22.0
Pork loin	3 oz.	20.0
Milk, whole	1 cup	9.0
Beans, red kidney	½ cup	7.5
Cheese, processed	1 oz.	7.0
Egg	1 med.	6.0
Lima beans	½ cup	6.0
Bacon	2 slices	5.0
Peanut butter	1 tbsp.	4.0
Ice cream	¼ pint	3.0
Potato	1 med.	3.0
Oatmeal	½ cup	2.5
Broccoli	½ cup	2.5
Bread, whole wheat	1 slice	2.0
Green beans	½ cup	1.0
Lettuce, head	½ cup	0.6
Orange juice	4 oz.	0.5

Water

Definitely the most underrated nutrient is water. In fact, you probably never even thought of it as a nutrient! Those eight glasses of water a day you've been told to drink are truly necessary for efficient bodily function.

I wouldn't be surprised if you've fallen victim to Madison Avenue advertising here, too—you *don't* need gallons of special "electrolyte replacement" drinks to fill your fluid needs when exercising. Most experts feel that plain old water, chilled because it's absorbed faster that way, is all you need before, during, and after exercise. There's very little strong evidence that commercial sport drinks help you perform better or recover faster than water.

How much to drink? At least 30 minutes before exercise, about 16 ounces of cold water. During exercise in the heat, about four to six ounces every 10–15 minutes. After exercise, be prudent with the amount you drink. Remember that the stomach can only absorb about 26 ounces per hour, so don't gulp

down much more than the recommended amounts.

Finally, sugar in fluids *slows* gastric emptying, the amount of time it takes to leave your stomach. Want to get fluids to your body as soon as possible? If you insist on a commercial drink, dilute it according to the instructions on pages 26–27. The *smartest* idea is to stick with plain H_2O.

GUIDELINES FOR ELECTROLYTE AND FLUID REPLACEMENT

Forget commercial hype, the following guidelines were set—based upon solid, scientific research—by four sports nutritionists.*

- To promote rapid absorption of fluid, beverages should contain, per quart, less than 25 grams of carbohydrate (two tablespoons sugar), less than 230 milligrams of sodium (one-tenth teaspoon of table salt), and less than 195 milligrams of potassium. They should contain *no* protein or fat. *Best temperature for absorption is 45°–55°F.*
- **Before exercise:** drink about 16 ounces of water 10–15 minutes beforehand.
- **During exercise:** drink 4–6 ounces of water at 10–15 minute intervals.
- **After exercise:** replace each pound of water lost with 16 oz. of water or the beverages listed below.
- **Master list of beverages for fluid replacement:** dilute commercial preparations as instructed below. *Most are far too concentrated according to researchers.*

Water—use as is. The *number one* choice.
Body Punch—1 part Body Punch/1 part water
E.R.G.—1 part E.R.G./1 part water
Bike Half-Time Punch—1 part Bike/2 parts water
Gatorade—1 part Gatorade/2 parts water
Quick Kick—1 part Quick Kick/2 parts water
Sportade—1 part Sportade/3 parts water
Take 5—1 part Take 5/7 parts water
Fruit Juices—1 part juice/7 parts water
Club Soda—use as is *if defizzed for* before/during use

Perrier—use as is *if defizzed for*
before/during use
Diet Sodas—1 part diet soda/1 part
water; defizz if for
before or during
exercise use
Sweetened Sodas—1 part soda/3 parts
water; defizz if used
before or during
exercise

* **Avoid or use with caution:** Alcohol and caffeine. Both promote urination and can be dehydrating; individual reactions vary widely.
* **Avoid completely:** *Salt tablets* interfere with fluid absorption, *aggravate* dehydration, and can cause nausea and stomach distress.

*From: *A Guide for Rapid Fluid and Safe Salt Replacement in Exercise.* Merle Best, Diana Galandak, Marilyn Schorin, and Frances Trakis-Fischer. Produced by EIC-NW, Morris Plains, New Jersey.

Vitamins and Minerals

Beware of more advertising hype. You've been sold another bill of goods here. No scientist in any reputable laboratory has ever shown that those huge doses you've been told to take actually work. You may be slightly deficient in one or more of the essential vitamins and minerals, but most experts recommend one multi-vitamin/mineral supplement a day to cover this possibility.

We Americans have become nothing more than brief way stations between health food store shelves and toilets. Most of the vitamins, minerals, and enzymes we take end up flushed away. The only exceptions to what I call the *Toilet Bowl Law* is the fat-soluble vitamins (A, D, E, and K) which can be stored (unlike the others), and can build up in *deadly* amounts.

An intelligent choice of foods from the basic groups, careful preparation, and one multi-supplement a day will fully meet the needs of any healthy person, athlete or not.

Save yourself a few bucks and try it next week. Forget the supplements, eat right, and psyche yourself up for a pill-free existence. It's risk free. I promise to let you go back to the stuff if you *really* need it. But give it a try.

METABOLISM: UNDERSTANDING WEIGHT CONTROL

Don't you hate that friend of yours who dines each night on two 17-inch pizzas, washes them down with a six-pack of Budweiser, and *loses* weight? Do you gain weight when just walking by a bakery? While the number of calories you burn through exercise obviously makes a difference, it often all boils down to one thing: metabolism.

Basal Metabolic Rate

Your *basal metabolic rate* (BMR) is the number of calories your body will burn in a state of absolute rest. Adding the calories you burn through activity and exercise gives you *total daily caloric expenditure.* The range of BMRs that you will find in a healthy, adult population is staggering. Most importantly, BMR can and *does* change with exercise and diet, sometimes going from bad to worse. Here's how to take charge.

If you're a healthy male in your twenties or early thirties, your BMR will likely be in the 1,600–2,000-calorie-per-day range. Females should adjust this number downward by 10%–20% due to their lower total muscle mass. Since muscles burn calories just sitting around, a lean, muscular person may burn more calories at rest than an obese person during light exercise! This is a major contribution of Nautilus to weight control: every pound of muscle you add raises your BMR and pushes you closer to two-pizza heaven.

Balancing the good news that BMR can be raised by adding muscle is the *very* bad news that it can be lowered through low-calorie diets.

Your body has evolved as a survival machine. It has "learned" to quickly adapt to periods of poor nutrition and low calorie intake. The brain structures that set BMR don't care *what* you look like in a mirror, they're far more concerned about keeping your bodily functions going. When you cut back on calories, adjustments are rapidly made so that operations can go on as usual with *less calories* taken in. No kidding here folks—you can drop your BMR as low as 700 calories a day by going on a very low calorie diet!

Let's say that when you started that diet two weeks ago your BMR was 2,000 a day, and the 330 calories you drank over three meals helped you lose a pound every two days (1,700 calories × two equals roughly 3,500 calories, or one pound). Now, two weeks later, you're still taking in 330 a day, but your BMR has dropped to 700. The difference between that and caloric intake is down to 370 a day from *1,670*. The body refuses to lose weight as quickly as it did. It'll take *nine* days to lose a pound now, not *two*. What do you do? Give up. Go back to 2,000 calories of food daily and guess what? Your BMR is still at 700, and you have a 1,300 calorie *surplus* each day. Back comes the weight.

This process is no fable. It has been documented clinically worldwide. Very-low calorie diets should *only* be used in hopelessly obese, hospital-bound patients. If you simply add about 200 calories of exercise to your day, and cut back 200 calories on food intake, you'll find lifetime weight control free and well within your grasp. Talk about an offer you can't refuse!

As for exercise's role in weight control, that 200 calories should best come from a daily, thirty-minute aerobics break. The old standbys are clearly the best, and they're all there in Chapter 11. You should also look for ways to burn up extra calories wherever possible: walk to work, park at the far end of the parking lot, get off your bus a few stops early, climb a few stairs. *It really works, I'm not kidding!* Expect your aerobic activities to burn anywhere from 250 (slow walking) to 800 (running, cross-country skiing) calories an hour.

Assessing BMR and Body Composition

For maximum efficiency in training, basal metabolic rate and body composition are critical numbers. Since the number of calories burned during exercise can be accurately estimated from tables, knowledge of BMR would allow you to compute your daily ca-

loric needs within very narrow limits. With the chances for under- or overeating thus reduced, weight control becomes a much easier process. Similarly, since body composition assessment can tell you whether fat or muscle tissue is being lost or gained, adjustments in training and/or diet can be made swiftly and accurately.

BMR is best measured by calculating the amount of oxygen you consume at total rest. Since each liter is burned with five calories of energy, your 24-hour BMR can be easily computed from a one-hour test. An alternate method requires that you compute the surface area of your body, then plug that number into a second equation.

My general feeling is that most people have a relatively good idea of the calories they can eat to maintain weight. With a little experimentation in diet and exercise, anyone can establish a steady weight without resorting to BMR assessment.

Similarly, while the concept of body composition assessment is critical, you can really do quite well with an old-fashioned, good, hard look in the mirror. If your Nautilus center *can* provide body composition measurements, so much the better.

The idea behind muscle/fat assessment is that what you weigh on a scale tells you nothing about what's inside. Eat too much after your Nautilus workouts and half of that six-pound gain might be fat. Eat right and all six might be muscle. Exercise too little while dieting and half of the weight lost will be muscle. Exercise and reduce calories and you'll lose mostly fat. I've tested countless men and women whose body weights showed absolutely no changes with training, but who had simultaneously lost fat and gained muscle for a net difference of zero. Oh, but the gains in health and fitness!

The most common method of assessment is the skinfold technique, where three to five pinches of skin and fat are taken from various sites on the body. If done by a trained technician, and plugged into the right equation (one for your age and sex), the results should be quite accurate. The technique all others are based on, however, is "hydrostatic" (underwater) weighing. This requires that you submerge yourself fully and expel all your air. What you weigh thus submerged is compared with what you weigh on dry land. With a knowledge of your "residual lung volume"—the amount of air left in your lungs after you blow everything you can out voluntarily—you can get a super-accurate measure of the fat percentage of your body. College-age males average about 14%, while females of the same age average about 24%. This difference is largely hormonal, and doesn't reduce greatly even with athletic training. Male marathoners may get as low as 3%, but females rarely drop below 12%. Cheer up, ladies—this difference makes you more efficient swimmers! Due to the added buoyancy, women burn about 30% fewer calories than men at any given speed. It also means that they can swim faster given the same number of calories expended. Someday you'll see women beat men heads-up in distance swimming.

NUTRITION FOR LIVING

When to Eat

Yes, when to eat makes a *big* difference. First off, your body treats one 2,000-calorie meal *very* differently than 2,000 calories split into three or four meals. Researchers have shown that even though your daily caloric expenditure may be 2,000, a single meal of that size can cause you to gain fat. Smaller meals, with the same number of calories divided up evenly, have no such effect. Think of trying to fill a bathtub faster than it can drain. It can take 700 calories at a time, but if it sees 2,000 at once, the overflow gets shunted off to be stored as fat.

DO'S AND DON'TS OF THE PRE-GAME MEAL*

The aim of the pre-game meal is to avoid discomfort or interference during the event from digestion. Optimal nutrition is a process that occurs in the weeks or months leading to the game,

not in the last meal beforehand. Special game-day precautions are necessary because pre-game excitement and anxiety may slow digestion and cause stomach upset.

Eating 3–4½ hours before strenuous exercise allows time for digestion and absorption but is not so early that feelings of hunger develop. Liquid meals that are low in fat and protein may be taken safely as close as two hours pre-game, but many athletes handle the drinks well within 30 minutes of game time.

Do

- Eat mostly carbohydrate foods, because they are more quickly digested and absorbed than high-fat or protein foods.
- Include two to three cups of liquid. Plain water can and should (in the heat) be consumed right up to game time.
- Eat a light meal with moderate portions. Don't overeat!
- Drink skim milk rather than whole milk.
- Remember that each athlete is unique and that optimal pre-game nutrition may require some experimentation.

Don't

- Eat fatty foods, such as heavily marbled meats or fried foods, since excessive fat slows stomach emptying.
- Eat high protein foods. Avoid protein supplements. Large quantities of protein will increase the need to urinate.
- Eat beans, cabbage, onions, cauliflower, etc., which can cause intestinal discomfort. If a food generally causes gas pains, avoid it.
- Eat or drink concentrated sugar foods and beverages closer than one hour before competition. They draw fluid *into* the gastrointestinal tract, which may result in cramps and nausea. Even worse, sugar stimulates insulin secretion, which, when combined with exercise, can result in low blood sugar and reduced endurance.
- Try a new food that you are not sure about in the meal before the event.

Good high-carbo choices: Breads, cereals, pancakes, pasta, rice, grains, beans, peas, lentils, fruits, vegetables, potatoes, soups.

*Adapted from The Pre-Event Meal by Merle Best, Diana Galandak, Marilyn D. Schorin, and Francis Trakis-Fischer; permission of New Jersey State Department of Education.

Second, you are better off eating the bulk of your calories during daytime hours when you're active and BMR is high. Third, treat breakfast as a major meal. It really *does* improve mental and physical function through the morning.

Finally, if you're wondering about eating before exercise or competition, skip the slow-to-digest fried and fatty foods and meat. Stick to complex carbos like pasta, and leave at least two hours for digestion. A big meal takes at least four hours to digest, but can stretch out way beyond that as well. If you must eat and run, the commercially available liquid meals are usually well-tolerated within 30 minutes of exercise.

What to Eat

The following advice is based on a major project by the National Academy of Sciences. It provides you with all required nutrients and about 1,800 calories a day. If your caloric needs vary, adjust accordingly. Don't forget that added exercise is the same thing as reduced calories taken in. If you can't get fresh vegetables and fruit, and can't or won't follow the advice given below on cooking and preparation, a multi-vitamin/mineral supplement couldn't hurt.

Fruits and Vegetables

Eat six or more daily servings of fruits and vegetables. A serving is one piece of fresh fruit or ½ cup frozen, raw, or cooked vegetables.

Fruits and vegetables high in vitamin C and/or A: mango, papaya, cantaloupe, watermelon, strawberries, citrus fruits, broccoli, spinach, kale, escarole, romaine lettuce, parsley, peppers, cabbage, white potatoes, sweet potatoes, carrots, acorn and butternut squash, and Brussels sprouts.

Of the recommended *cruciferous* vegetables—broccoli, Brussels sprouts, kale, cabbage, and cauliflower—only cauliflower is not high in vitamins A or C.

Whole Grains and Cereals

Eat five servings of whole grains. Two slices of bread, two muffins, or ½ cup of cooked cereal equals one serving. Whole grain products include whole wheat bread, brown rice, corn, cornmeal, wheat germ, bran, barley, buckwheat groats, bulgur, and oatmeal.

Protein-Rich Foods

Eat two to three servings of low-fat dairy products, lean fish, meat, poultry, eggs, beans, or nuts. A cup of skim milk, 1½ ounces of cheese, or a cup of low-fat yogurt equals one serving. Dairy products high in fat are whole-milk products, cream, most cheeses (harder cheeses are better than soft), ice cream, and sour cream.

Two or three ounces of boneless fish, meat, or poultry or one egg equals one serving. Trim exterior fat from meat; choose meat with little marbling; eat white meat chicken and turkey and remove skin.

Up to a cup of cooked beans or ¼ cup of nuts equals one serving. The dried-beans category includes lentils, dried peas, and chickpeas. Nuts are also high in fat.

Occasional Inclusions

In addition to oil, butter, and margarine, foods high in fat include mayonnaise, salad dressing, rich desserts, and fried and creamed dishes.

Tips on Preparation and Cooking

Here are some helpful/healthful tips you can take to the market and kitchen:

- Stress complex carbohydrates. At least 60% of your daily calories should come from carbos, and 75% of that amount should be from the complex forms.
- Protein is almost always overconsumed. Protein calories should total about 10%–15% of your daily intake.
- One serving of liver per week will give you a two-week supply of vitamin B_{12}, a 10-day

SAMPLE REDUCED-CALORIE DIET PLANS

The following four daily plans provide approximately 1,200 calories and a full complement of essential nutrients (don't forget your eight glasses of water!). It is unwise for a healthy, exercising adult to go far below the 1,200 calories limit. Remember that your metabolism will slow as you reduce calories—exercise and calorie control work best when used together.

Breakfast	Lunch	Dinner
6 oz. fruit juice or fruit ½ cup bran cereal with raisins ½ cup skim milk 1 slice whole wheat bread or bran-fruit muffin 1 cup coffee/tea	1 cup tuna salad 1–2 tbsp. dressing Celery, cucumber, tomato (½) 2 melba toast or 1 slice whole wheat bread 1 apple	Salad: lettuce, spinach, tomato, raw vegetables, 1 tsp. vinegar dressing 4 oz. cooked meat—lean meat, poultry, fish 1 medium baked potato 1 fruit
4 oz. stewed prunes 3/4 cup cooked cereal 1 cup skim milk for cereal or drink	1 cup lentil soup or broth ½ cup low-fat cottage cheese 1 carrot ½ small cucumber ½ tomato 3 melba toast 1 small orange	4 oz. grapefruit juice 5 oz. broiled salmon cooked with margarine ½ cup brown rice ½ cup cooked spinach or small salad
4 oz. orange juice ¾ cup shredded wheat 1 cup skim milk 1 cup coffee/tea	1 cup vegetable–barley soup 2 tbsp. peanut butter and jelly (each) 2 slices grain bread ¼ cantaloupe	2 egg mushroom omelet (margarine) ½ whole wheat roll 1½ cups mixed green salad with raw vegetables 1 cup plain yogurt with 1 small banana
1 cup plain yogurt with ½ apple and 1 tbsp. raisins 1 slice whole wheat toast 1 tsp. margarine 1 cup coffee/tea	1½ cups tomato soup Chicken sandwich with 2 oz. chicken, 2 tsp. mayonnaise, 2 slices whole grain bread 5 medium asparagus spears 1 medium tangerine	4 oz. vegetable juice 4 oz. lean meat or fish 1 small baked potato 1 medium stalk broccoli 1 tsp. margarine ½ medium grapefruit

Unlimited amounts of diet beverages may be consumed.

---

supply of vitamin A, a two-day supply of riboflavin, and 12% of your daily iron needs.

- Lean meats, skinless poultry, and low-fat dairy products offer more nutrients per calorie than their fattier versions and may reduce the risk of diet-induced cancers.
- Whole grains (whole wheat pasta, oatmeal, brown rice) have more nutrients than foods made from refined grains (even if enriched).

- Dark-green, leafy vegetables and deep-yellow vegetables have more vitamin A than lighter-colored ones.
- Fresh or frozen fruits and vegetables are more nutrient-packed than canned ones. If fresh foods have been long in transit or storage, the frozen type may be more nutritious.
- Look for produce that has been kept cold in the store. This reduces the effects of nutrient-destroying enzymes.

- Fruits ripened on the plant and in the sun have more vitamin C than those picked green. Outdoor-grown tomatoes have twice the vitamin C of greenhouse versions.
- Ripe fruits and vegetables should be stored cold until eaten.
- Potatoes, canned foods, and grain foods should be stored in a cool, dark, and dry place. Don't refrigerate potatoes.
- Milk and bread should be kept in opaque containers to prevent destruction of riboflavin and vitamins A and D.

- Wash produce quickly, for soaking can rinse away water-soluble vitamins and minerals
- Refrigerate all cooked foods that are not going to be eaten immediately.
- Keep fresh, cut, and cooked foods well-wrapped to reduce exposure to air.
- Waterless cooking, pressure cooking, steaming, stir-frying, and microwaving are least destructive of nutrients.
- Reduce cooking time as well as the surface area of food exposed during cooking wherever possible.

5

THE NAUTILUS OPERATING MANUAL: PRINCIPLES OF DESIGN

What is it that makes Nautilus special? Why have over 2,000 fitness centers and countless amateur and professional athletic teams, hospitals, rehabilitation centers, and corporations made Nautilus the cornerstone of their strength programs? It surely isn't advertising or marketing dollars. No multimillion-dollar Madison Avenue ad campaigns for Nautilus Sports/Medical Industries! No payoffs to big-name athletes who couldn't even tell Nautilus from a barbell. No, plain and simple, Nautilus *works*. In less time than anything else. But, you ask, HOW? That's what this chapter is all about.

STRENGTH-TRAINING FEATURES

In designing the ideal strength-training machine, consideration must be given to how the body works and how strength is developed. We can identify *eight* features of Nautilus equipment that address these two issues. It is in having *all eight* that Nautilus became the generic term for strength-training equipment. They are:

- variable resistance
- direct resistance
- rotary resistance
- positive *and* negative work
- resistance in the position of full contraction
- unlimited speed of movement
- preexhaustion principle

Let's look at them one by one.

Variable Resistance

We saw in Chapter 3 that each muscle in your body has its own, unique strength curve, the amount of force it can create as it moves through its working range. This changing strength capability is explained by two factors: the internal arrangement of muscle fibers and the way the muscle attaches to or "inserts on" its target bone.

These strength curves can be *very* different, even in muscles that appear to do related things. For example, the four quadriceps muscles extend (kick out) your lower leg, and have a strength curve that looks like an inverted letter U. In contrast, the three hamstrings muscles flex (pull back) your lower leg, but have a strength curve that starts high but gets progressively weaker as you flex.

We also saw in Chapter 3 that the true resistance of a barbell, which is called torque, itself changes as your muscles lift the weight. Unfortunately, *this* pattern can only *by chance* match the pattern of the lifting muscle's strength curve. The mismatch means one thing: *inefficiency*.

The ideal strength-training device should be able to change the effective resistance on the muscle *in the same way* that the muscle changes. If the muscle gets stronger then weaker as it contracts, the resistance should get heavier then lighter. If the muscle gets progressively weaker as it contracts, the resistance should get progressively smaller.

What our ideal device is trying to do is keep the muscle working at high intensity through its full range of motion. Thanks to the use of an ingenious, off-round pulley called a *cam*, Nautilus can do that.

The cam makes Nautilus a *variable resistance device*. Better still, let's call it an *accurate* variable resistance device. We should not forget that barbells are *also* variable resistance devices, the difference being that the variation is random and not scientifically designed!

How does the cam work? Since the distance from the cam's *axis of rotation* to the point at which the *chain leaves the pulley groove* varies, the laws of physics dictate that the torque or turning force must change. The cam on each Nautilus machine is shaped to mimic the strength curve of the muscle(s) being trained. Need a heavy load at 121° because your muscle is strong at that point? No problem—the radius of the cam will be long. Need a light load at 73°? Just shorten the radius accordingly.

Critics and competitors of Nautilus often argue that not everyone's biceps strength curve is identical, and that cams are therefore useless. It just ain't so—or at least the latter part isn't. There *are* minor differences among people, but the basic strength curves are similar enough to allow one cam to work for just about everybody on each machine.

Direct Resistance

Ever heard the expression, "A chain is only as strong as its weakest link"? If 99 of its 100 links can withstand 1,000 pounds of force, but the 100th only ten, then the chain will break if given eleven. You may never have realized it before, but many strength-training machines and strength exercises suffer from the same problem.

Take the case of chin-ups, a wonderful exercise that primarily trains the *latissimus dorsi* of your back. Grip the bar, pull yourself up slowly, then lower slowly. What muscles besides the latissimus (the "lats") were working? Why, the gripping muscles of the forearm and the biceps and brachialis in the upper arm, of course. This can be a *major* problem if you have either well-developed lats or particularly weak forearms or upper arms. Many women cannot do a single chin-up because their grip strength is insufficient. Many advanced strength athletes are forced to stop chinning prematurely (their lats still going strong) because their grips or upper arms fail.

This leads to our "weak link in the chain" theory of strength training. In order to fully and efficiently train a muscle, weak links in the chain must be eliminated. If a major muscle like the lats must be trained through *other* muscles, failure of these smaller and weaker "links" will reduce the training effect on the larger muscle. The solution: Direct resistance.

Wherever possible, Nautilus designers have attempted to let the target muscle apply its force *directly* to the machine. Want to skip chin-ups? Try the Nautilus Pullover machine. Since the lats attach to the humerus (upper arm), the resistance in this machine is applied by the elbows. *No* grip problems. *No* biceps/brachialis involvement.

As we'll see at the end of this chapter, Nautilus has ingeniously turned the tables on the "weak link" problem by incorporating it into its Compound machines. Devilish idea!

Rotary Resistance

If you stop to think about it, all motion by the body is based on rotation at the joints. Sure, you can move your hand away from you in a straight line, but that movement is accomplished with rotation at the wrist, elbow, and shoulder. Any device attempting to optimally train a muscle should allow it to work in a natural movement pattern. Devices that don't allow rotary motion are simply inefficient.

While the machine must allow rotary movement, it must also allow the individual to align the axis of his joint rotation with its own mechanical axis. Try doing a biceps curl on a Nautilus machine with your elbow joint axes several inches from the cam axes. Not only is it inefficient, it hurts!

The best example of devices that don't offer perfect rotary resistance for every exercise is rowing machines. These do a generally fine job of letting you simulate rowing, but they just don't work for all the other things their manufacturers tell you they can do. Since the axes of joint and machine rotation cannot be aligned, the exercises are inefficient, uncomfortable (try one and see for yourself), and possibly dangerous.

Nautilus and most other popular machines these days offer rotary resistance.

Positive and Negative Work

As you may recall from Chapter 3, a muscle can contract either concentrically or eccentrically. When a muscle contracts and shortens, concentric or *positive* work is performed. When a muscle attempts to shorten but is lengthened by a greater force, eccentric or *negative* work is performed. Raising a weight overhead would involve shortening/concentric/positive work by the deltoids and triceps, while lowering it against gravity's pull would involve lengthening/eccentric/negative work by the same muscles.

Positive and negative work are *very* different chemically and mechanically. Because the cross-bridges are only slipping backward during negatives, the energy cost is *much* lower. In fact, the negative work of lowering a barbell requires 60%–70% less energy than the positive work of lifting it. This also partly explains why you can lower about 40% more weight than you can lift with any given muscle.

How do negatives fit into the weight-training picture? Manufacturers whose equipment doesn't allow negative work will tell you that they *don't* fit, but they're wrong. You should pay *strict* attention to the negative or lowering phase of every repetition on every exercise you do. Research has repeatedly shown that negatives can build strength and size as quickly, or even more quickly, than positives. By *combining* negatives and positives (details later . . .) you can double your results.

Stretching in the Starting Position

The old image of the muscle-bound weightlifter was no lie. Before the value of flexibility became more widely appreciated, lifters worked through short movements to build as much bulk as possible. By not working at the extremes of their ranges of motion (full flexion and extension) where they were the weakest, these lifters lost significant amounts of flexibility. If *you* play your cards right, though, you can have strength and flexibility at the same time.

Most Nautilus machines do at least a creditable job of stretching you in the starting position of the exercise. The best example is the Pullover machine, which can work your latissimus dorsi through as much as a 240° range of motion. Some Nautilus machines are better than others because anatomy doesn't always allow simultaneous strength and flexibility training. In any case, few manufacturers have done as good a job as Nautilus in taking your muscles through their full range of motion.

As I noted earlier, remember that permanent increases in flexibility come mostly from static (nonbouncing), prolonged stretching of a warm muscle, which Nautilus cannot do. Should your leisure time pursuits require more flexibility than you've got now, take a look at Chapter 12.

Resistance in the Position of Full Contraction

Since high-efficiency strength training requires that the muscle be stressed through its full range of motion, it would be silly to let the muscle rest at the end of its range. Unfortunately, many devices have this shortcoming. Either through poor design of the machine, or by using an exercise that lets the joint "lock out" (placing the load on the bones instead of the muscles), resistance in the position of full contraction is often lost.

Nautilus again scores high grades here. Through smart mechanical design and the use of exercises where you *can't* lock out, Nautilus has incorporated this exercise requirement into most of its machines.

Unlimited Speed of Movement

The speed at which your muscles move your limbs during strength training should not be limited. Small accelerations and decelerations are critical in allowing you to squeeze out that extra effort at the end of a set. They also make your strength work much more similar to real-world athletic efforts. Changes in speed and acceleration are seen in all sports, but constant velocity or "isokinetic" movements are strictly laboratory phenomena. Most strength experts see the unlimited speed of movement capability of Nautilus and barbells as a major advantage over isokinetics.

The Preexhaustion Principle

Nautilus is no longer alone in incorporating the first seven design features we've discussed into their machines. They are, however, the only manufacturer that gives you the Preexhaustion Principle. Does it make a difference!

Remember back to our weak-link-in-the-chain theory? And how I told you that Nautilus turned "bad news" into "good news"? This is how it's done: Our goal is super-high-intensity training of a muscle in one two-minute exercise (more on that later). We know that direct resistance is critical, because we don't want smaller muscles to fail before larger ones. So, our first 12–15 repetitions are on a machine that offers direct resistance. At the completion of this set, we've done all we could to overload the muscle. Unless we immediately begin a *second* exercise that lets the weaker links in the chain, rested from their inactivity during the first reps, help the major muscle go even further. What we've done is *preexhaust* the larger muscle, then train it still further with the help of the "weak links in the chain."

Using our original Pullover machine example, let's look at what would happen if we added a pulldown exercise to the Pullover machine frame. First we preexhaust the latissimus dorsi with the direct resistance offered by the Pullover. We then reach for the pulldown bar and begin that exercise. With the help of fresh and rested biceps and brachialis muscles, the lats are pushed closer to total exhaustion, and the last ounce of effort can be squeezed out. All in about two minutes. Let's call this machine the Pullover/Torso Arm combination. Good idea, because that's what Nautilus calls it!

Here's a list of the other Nautilus "Compound" machines that use the Preexhaustion Principle:

Machine	Order of Exercises
Compound Leg	Leg Extension then Leg Press
Behind Neck/Torso Arm	Behind Neck then Pulldown
Double Shoulder	Lateral Raise then Overhead Press
Double Chest	Arm Cross then Incline Press

These names Greek to you? Wait just one more chapter.

6

THE NAUTILUS OPERATING MANUAL: TRAINING RULES AND REGULATIONS

Nautilus truly stands alone when it comes to training theory. Abandon all thoughts of multiple sets and three-hour workouts—Nautilus training is *high quality* but *low quantity*. One set, taken to the point of momentary muscular failure, is felt to be sufficient stimulus for maximal growth. Not three sets. Not five sets. One. To failure.

GO TO FAILURE

I can't quote you dozens of laboratory studies proving that one high-quality set is superior to two or more sets. There aren't any such studies. (Neither are there studies proving the opposite.) We can't look to Nautilus for experimental data because they can't provide any. What *do* we have? Just *thousands* of testimonials and converts. People who, using their own or their athletes' bodies as laboratories, have found that one set, taken to momentary muscular failure, *is* enough. Enough for high school Junior Varsity squads. Enough for the pros.

The scientist in me wishes that there were loads of studies to quote, facts and figures to dazzle you. The realist in me knows that the only thing that will *convince* you is trying it for yourself.

Intensity—And One Set to Failure

If you're not training on Nautilus right now, chances are that you've been told that at least three sets are necessary for maximal muscular growth. Such advice is probably true for the equipment you're training on. Without the cam and the other design features we discussed in Chapter 5, you're using less-than-maximally-efficient machines. The combination of these features in Nautilus allows high intensity (quality) and a sizeable reduction in quantity.

The logic of Nautilus training is flawless: Start with the least amount of high-quality work possible (one set of 12–15 repetitions) then add more reps or sets if results are not forthcoming. If one set, taken to failure, isn't enough for you (unlikely if you follow my instructions), add a second set. It seems pretty dumb to me to start with three or four sets, and then never really know if you're over-working and wasting time. Unless you've got hours to burn in the weightroom, the one-set-to-failure idea makes great sense.

What is all this nonsense about going to failure, you ask? Simple—work as hard as you can and you'll never have to worry about guessing how hard 75%, or 90%, or 95% is. Just go to 100%—momentary muscular failure—the inability of the muscle to perform any further reps in good form. I'll skip all the scientific mumbo jumbo here and just ask you to follow the logic of it all. One brief but terribly intense set has worked for tens of thousands. Why waste your time with three or more sets if one will do? (If you *insist* on the scientific mumbo jumbo, read about re-cruitment of the FG fibers in Chapter 3. Going to failure will ensure that these babies are fully recruited and trained.)

How Many Reps?

Again, with no solid research to turn to, we're left with logic and experience. It seems a pretty solid bet that, given the efficiency of Nautilus equipment, most of you won't need to perform more than 15 repetitions on any one exercise. This does *not* mean that you quit whenever you complete your 15th rep. It means that you should select a weight that will allow you to complete only 15 reps, in perfect form, before reaching momentary muscular failure. If, on any particular day, you get to 15 and there's more steam in your engines, keep going. If your chosen weight can't be lifted more than eight times, lower the weight and try another set after a short rest. Try less weight next time.

The Nautilus Compound machines are something of an exception to this rule, since they combine two exercises and twice the number of reps. As always, experiment to find what works best for you. Many readers will obtain all the strength and size benefits they desire from just the first exercise on a compound machine. Advanced trainees will surely want to go for the double.

And speaking of you advanced trainees,

look what I've got for you: After your twelve positive/negative reps, we're going to do some very special negative variations. As will beginners, you'll start each exercise with 12–15 reps at a slow and controlled speed (more later). You should shoot for momentary mus-cular failure at 15, just like novices. Now, however, the fun starts. Optimally, you'll have a training partner or instructor to help with the negatives that follow what you *thought* was momentary muscular failure. You're not finished yet.

First up is *negative-only* exercise. Your partner/trainer will lift the weight or perform the concentric contraction for you; all you do is lower the weight. *Slowly.* To a count of ten. You'll do three or four of these before mov-ing on to *negative-emphasized* reps. Your trainer again performs the concentric lift, but now adds his own force to that of the weight stack while you resist its downward return. Talk about pain! Talk about results! There are no solid guidelines as to number of reps here, but don't expect to be able to do many more than three or four.

The advanced trainee then will shoot for the following:

12–15 positive/negative reps followed im-mediately by . . .

3–4 negative-only reps followed imme-diately by . . .

3–4 negative-emphasized reps.

Why is all this grief necessary? A little story here to explain why momentary muscular failure is not always easy to reach without extra help. I strength-trained the Miami Uni-versity of Ohio's Women's Swim Team over the winter break of 1981. They had come to swim in the Florida warmth, and we lucked into each other during swim practice. I of-fered them the use of the Nautilus weight-room/showroom and they went for it.

Looking around for a healthy demonstra-tor, I spied a tall, lean, athletic young woman (who turned out to be a two-time All-Ameri-can). I positioned her in the Pullover machine and began talking about momentary muscu-lar failure and the number of reps required to reach it. Boy, had I picked the right person! This young woman was a *worker.* She got to

15 reps and looked for all the world like she had truly reached momentary failure. I began the negative-only reps by doing the positive work and handing her the bar, expecting that she would be out of control and wiped out. Wrong. She smiled and did a perfect 15-second, negative-only rep. After three more of these, with what looked like 50 more reps left in her lats, we began the negative-emphasized reps. It took four of these to truly push her to momentary failure. The total: 15 positive/negative reps, 4 negative-only, 4 negative-emphasized. I had made my point to the team that failing at 15 reps isn't *true* momentary muscular failure.

True failure requires much more than most people are willing to give. Advanced trainees and elite athletes will tell you it's worth every ounce of effort, though. Incidentally, I received a wonderful card signed by the whole team about a month later, thanking me for the education and the training I provided. It wasn't a *total* coincidence that they won the Division II National Championships later that spring.

If you can't find a training partner or instructor, you've got an option on several machines called *negative-accentuated* exercise. On machines such as the Leg Extension, you can do negative-only reps on one leg at a time by lifting the weight with both but lowering with only one. The use of both arms or legs will give the single limb a heftier-than-usual load, which is fine—remember, a muscle can lower about 40% more weight than it can lift.

You can try negative-accentuated reps on any machine that won't throw you into a dangerous posture with only one limb working (like the Pullover machine). Use common sense here to avoid potential injury.

Some of the workouts listed in Chapter 10 include exercises that are entirely negative-only, -emphasized, or -accentuated. Advanced trainees should experiment with sets and whole workouts that include no positive work. Shoot for at least ten reps, and hold each for a count of ten. Either you or your trainer should count out loud as you lower the weight—it definitely helps.

How Fast the Reps?

"Slow and controlled" are the words to live by. That old Nautilus advice about two seconds up (positive lift) and four seconds down (negative lower) is pretty useless because some machines require three times more rotation than others. (Compare the Pullover machine, at 240°, with the Lateral Raise on the Double Shoulder machine, at about 80°.) As long as you *never* jerk or explode into the weights, or throw them so that they travel under their own momentum, you'll be fine.

The negative phase of every rep *should* be slower because the speed reduction "fools" the muscle into feeling a heavier load. Since you can lower more than you can lift, and it would be tough to add weight to the stack each time you lower it, the speed trick serves a useful purpose. And it works.

If you don't feel quite sure about recommended speed yet, here are some examples to take back to the machines:

Exercise	Recommended Speed for Concentric
Leg Extension	3 seconds/30° per sec
Pullover	4 seconds/50–60° per sec
Arm Cross (Double Chest)	3 seconds/30° per sec
Biceps Curl	3 seconds/45° per sec

This should give you a feel for what "slow and controlled" means.

Speed between Machines

Many of you won't have the option of choosing your workout speed. Crowded commercial facilities rarely allow you the luxury of setting seat heights and weight stacks in advance! Your best bet is to find the slack hours of your facility when fast circuits are more likely to work. In most places, mid-morning and mid-afternoon are the quietest times.

If you're after cardiovascular conditioning as well as strength, the "Express Circuit" is for you. Though the muscles being strength trained aren't receiving aerobic benefits, the heart and respiratory muscles are contracting rhythmically, repetitively, and at a high rate for 20 minutes. It is difficult to directly measure heart and lung benefits, but the probability is high that circuit training on Nautilus has a strong effect. Nautilus doesn't replace aerobic exercise, but it helps.

If you're after pure, unadulterated strength, take your time between machines. The stress of circuit training reduces the amount of effort you can put into each exercise, which will in turn reduce your results. I advise a minimum of three minutes between machines, and don't be afraid to stretch or shake out a bit if you tighten up.

How Often?

You gluttons for punishment will absolutely hate this—high-quality Nautilus work will get you as big and strong as you want on two workouts a week. Employees at Nautilus have access to a private and well-equipped gym which doubles as a showroom. During the quiet hours of the day, trainers and their victims saunter in, set all the seat heights, set all the weight stacks, and get to work. These brutally-hard, rapid-fire workouts last no more than 20 minutes and rarely occur more than twice a week, because (a) that's all you need and (b) that's all you can handle. I personally fell asleep and cracked my head into my desk three times on off-days because three of these workouts a week was too much. Cutting back to two-a-week solved the problem and didn't reduce my training gains one iota.

If you have a partner/trainer and can do negatives after each set, try two a week and see if it works for you. Under no circumstances should anyone train more than three times a week, and workouts should be spaced at least 48 hours apart. Split routines (upper body on day one, lower on day two, upper on day three, etc.) are *not* recommended. You'll be constantly tearing down your body and

getting less results than if you give yourself time to recover and rebuild. Again, try it and see.

THE FOURTEEN COMMANDMENTS

1. Perform only one set of four to six exercises for the lower body and six to eight exercises for the upper body. Vary this if your sport involves disproportionate use of the lower body. Compound machines count as *two* exercises. You should do no more than 14 *exercises,* not machines.

2. Select your weight load so that you will reach failure in anywhere from 12–15 reps. If you're just starting out, the first six workouts (two weeks) should use very light weights, and you *should not* try to go to failure.

3. Continue each exercise to the point of momentary muscular failure, that is, when no additional reps can be completed in good form. If you reach 15 reps with good form in *two* consecutive workouts, increase the weight 5% for your next workout.

4. *Never* rest the weights upon the weight stack between reps. Remember the phrase "touch and go." This will remind you to touch the weights upon the stack *briefly* then *go!*

5. Always work the larger muscles first. Beginning with the smaller muscles can lead to overall fatigue before the more important major muscles have been trained. The proper training sequences are presented in Chapter 10.

6. Concentrate on flexibility by letting the machines *slowly* draw you into the stretched starting position. *Permanent* gains in flexibility will only come through static stretching, but letting the machine stretch you will improve the range of motion through which you develop usable strength.

7. Accentuate the lowering or negative phase of every repetition. Follow the guidelines given earlier in this chapter on the use of negative-emphasized, -accentuated, and -only after the first 12–15 reps of a set.

8. Move slower, not faster, if ever in doubt about speed. No movement should be com-

pleted in *less* than two seconds. Do *not* throw the weights or explode into them. This is both dangerous and nonproductive.

9. If strength gains are to be maximized, rest for several minutes between machines. If cardiovascular gains are to be maximized, move as quickly as possible between machines. Working out at a slow hour at your facility will help.

10. *Always breathe normally.* Holding your breath immediately shuts down the return of blood to your heart and can literally kill you. Research has shown that blood pressure can exceed 300 over 200 (systolic/diastolic) during the performance of a maximal lift with the breath held! (Normal is 115/75.)

11. Constantly strive for increasing the amount of weight that can be lifted 15 times with perfect form. Stagnating at a particular weight will obviously reduce results. *Never* sacrifice form, however, in the attempt for more reps.

12. Train no more than three times a week. Leave at least 48 hours between workouts. If you can work with a training partner, and can handle the extra intensity, experiment with two workouts a week. If you find yourself fatigued or progressing more slowly than expected, *reduce* your work load. *Do not overwork.*

13. Keep accurate records. Seat height should be set at your first workout. Note on a card each day's weight, reps, and negative variations. Training logs for Nautilus are also available.

14. Vary your workouts often. Refer to Chapter 10 for a list of routines that you can use or modify as you like.

7
THE LOWER BODY

The following three chapters bring you what you've been waiting for. Each chapter will be preceded by a list of muscle groups and the machines that can be used to train them.

Use this book at your fitness center. Don't expect to memorize the training details at home then jump right into a perfect workout at the gym. The correct use of these machines is not always obvious, and results will suffer if you don't start out by doing it right!

Your workouts will generally start with the lower body, since large muscle groups should be trained before small. For variation (see Chapter 10), workouts *can* be started with the upper body.

Okay, here we go:

Muscle Groups	Nautilus® Machine
Hip Extensors	
Gluteus maximus, hamstrings	Duo Squat, Hip and Back, Leg Curl
Hip Flexors	
Rectus femoris of the quadriceps group, iliopsoas	Hip Flexor, Leg Extension

Muscle Groups	Nautilus® Machine
Quadriceps	
Vastus lateralis, medialis, intermedius; rectus femoris	Duo Squat, Leg Extension, Compound Leg
Hamstrings	
Semimembranosus, Semitendinosus, Biceps Femoris	Duo Squat, Leg Curl, Hip and Back
Adductors	
Adductor longus, brevis; gracilis	Adductor Machine
Abductors	
Gluteus medius, minimus; Tensor Fascia Latae	Abductor Machine
Ankle Extensors	
Gastrocnemius; Soleus	Calf Raise (Multi-Exercise)
Ankle Flexors	
Tibialis Anterior	Foot Flexion (Leg Curl)

THE HIP AND BACK MACHINE

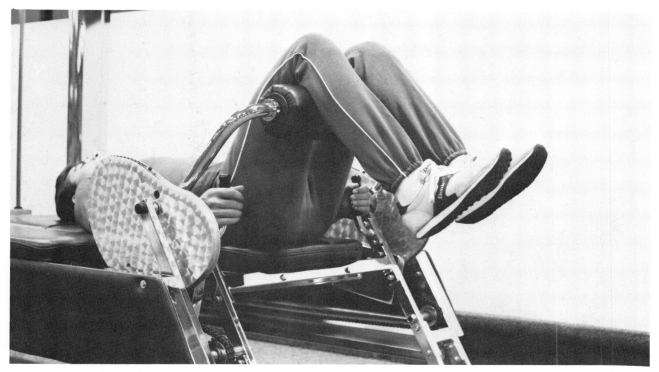

1. Slide onto pad from either side and place both legs over the rollers.

2. Arms are extended, grip open; hip joint should roughly match the cam's rotation axis.

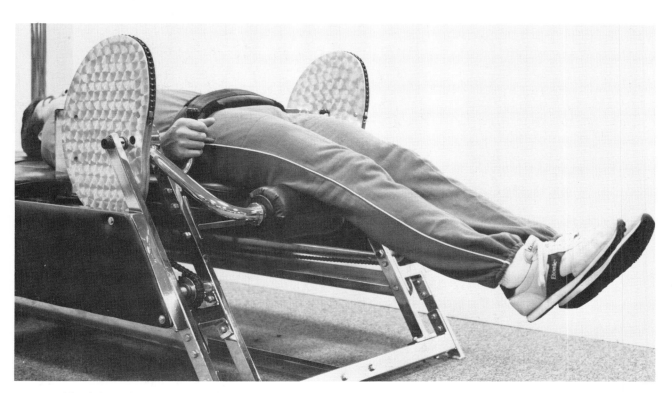

1. Extend both legs slowly and completely. DO NOT arch back by extending beyond 180°–190°. Hold this position for a count of two.

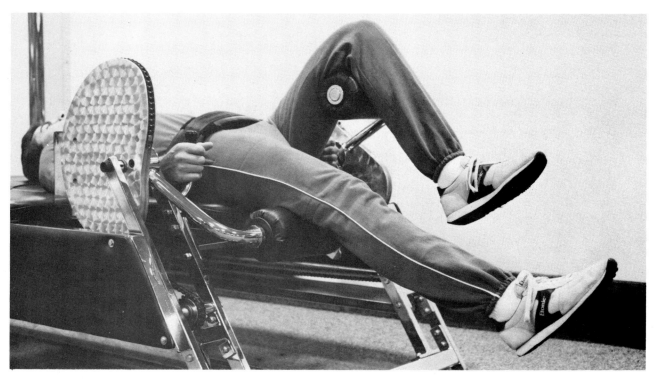

1. Holding one leg perfectly steady, let the other leg rise toward the torso.

2. As the leg raises, let the lower leg flex backward to form about a 90° angle with the back of the thigh.

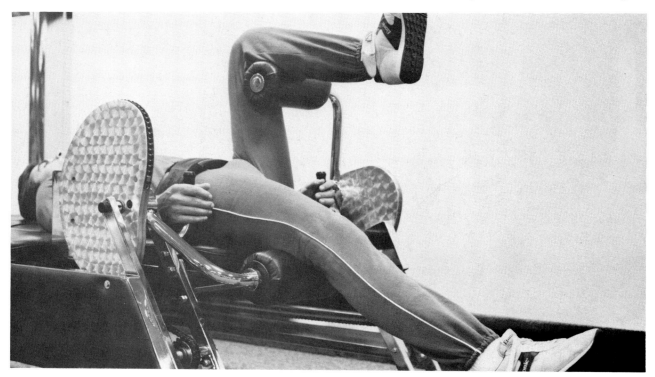

1. At full flexion of the leg on the torso, and keeping the down leg motionless, return the up leg to its starting position.
2. *Do not* extend the up foot toward the ceiling. Your return to starting position (hip extension) should exactly mimic the hip flexion movement.
3. Pause for a count of two in the fully extended position. Do not arch the back.
4. Repeat with the opposite leg.

THE DUO SQUAT MACHINE

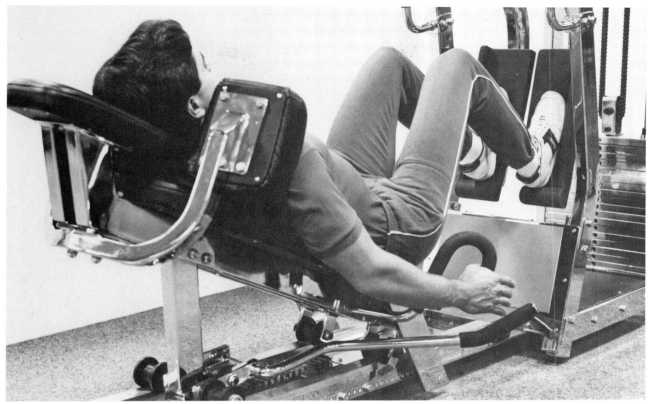

1. Seat position can only be set from inside the machine through trial and error.
2. Climb in and push yourself firmly up into the shoulder pads. Maintain an open grip.
3. Place both feet onto the foot pedals at the lowest position.

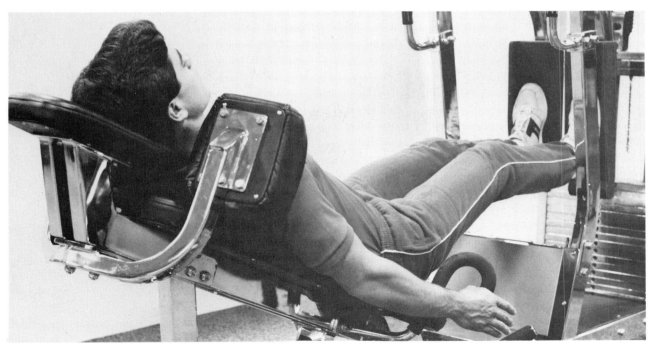

1. Push out slowly until you either extend the legs fully or reach the crossbar (next photo). Correct seat position will not allow you to extend the legs fully.

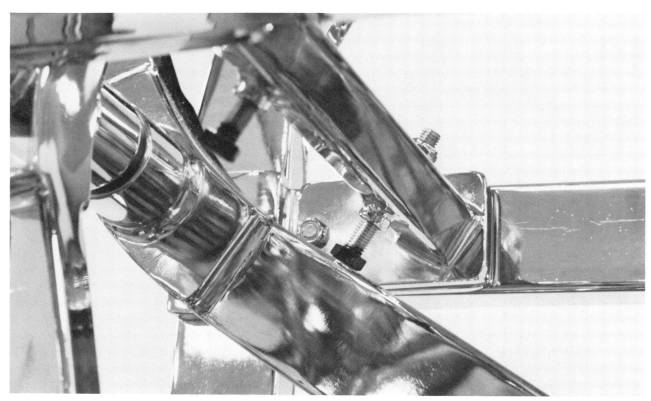

1. Locate the crossbar with the two bolts and set your seat position so the machine's levers meet these bolts when your legs are extended to 160°–170°.

2. If you can extend your legs fully before the levers reach the bolts, move the seat closer.

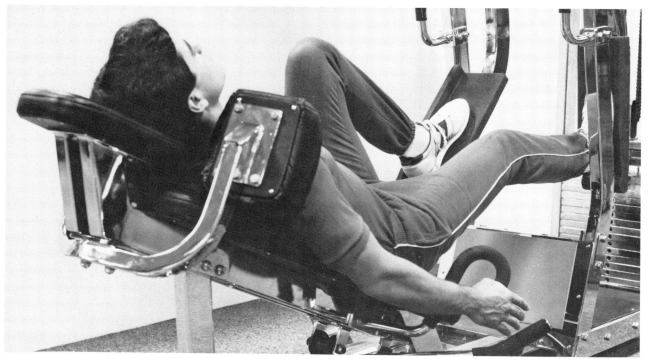

1. Now you're ready to go. With both legs extended, keep one motionless and let the other flex slowly backward toward the torso.

2. Get as full a flexion as possible, then slowly extend outward toward the other leg.

3. Hold this position and repeat with the opposite leg.

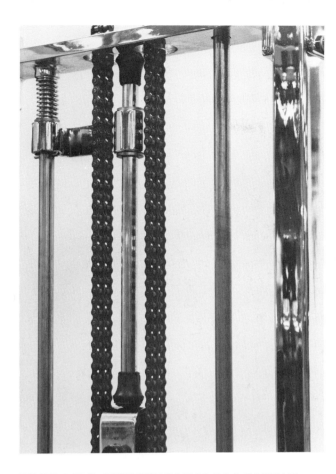

1. The infimetric bar can be swung into position between the chains and above the weight stack.
2. Infimetric or Akinetic training requires that you extend both legs simultaneously until the weight stack presses the infimetric bar against the cross-member.
3. Slowly extend one leg while resisting and flexing with the other. Do not let the weight stack drop off the infimetric bar.
4. Reverse movements by extending the flexed leg and resisting with the opposite.
5. Nautilus has arbitrarily called this exercise *Infimetric* if you do it with zero or one plate, and *Akinetic* if you use more than one plate. Don't ask why.

THE LEG EXTENSION MACHINE

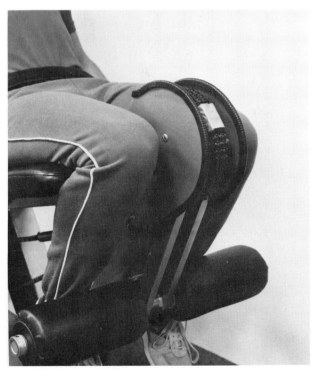

1. If your machine has an adjustable seat back, position it so that your knees align with the machine's axis of rotation.

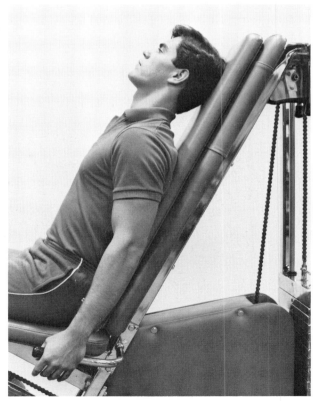

1. On a nonadjustable-seat leg extension, you may require one long back pad to move you forward into the correct position.

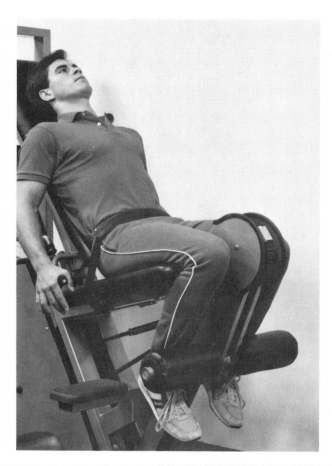

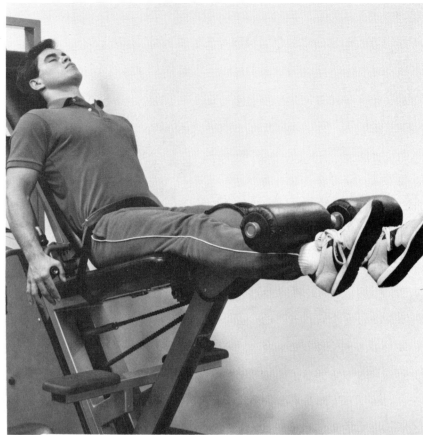

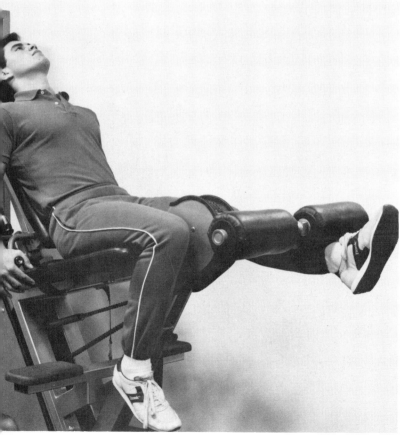

Above, left:
1. You may find it easiest to place your feet behind the rollers before sitting back.
2. With an open grip and the head and torso relaxed against the back pad, assume the starting position.

Above, right:
1. Extend both legs slowly to 180° and hold this position for a count of two.
2. Return both legs simultaneously but do not rest the weight stack upon full flexion. If your weight load does reach the rest of the stack, touch down briefly and go. I call this "touch and go."

Below, left:
1. You may do unilateral (one-leg) negatives by extending with both legs then dropping one off and lowering with the other. This is called "negative-accentuated exercise."

THE COMPOUND LEG MACHINE

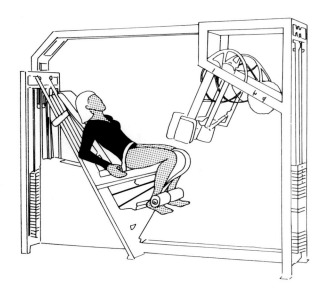

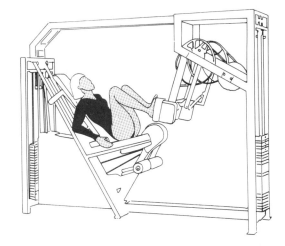

1. Perform the leg extension exercise as above.

1. Swing the foot pads down into position for the squat.
2. Move the seat forward to give you a more complete range of motion. If you have knee problems, do not move the seat forward.
3. Keeping an open grip and the head and torso back and relaxed, extend out slowly to just short of the 180° position.
4. Hold for a count of two and return slowly.

THE LEG CURL MACHINE

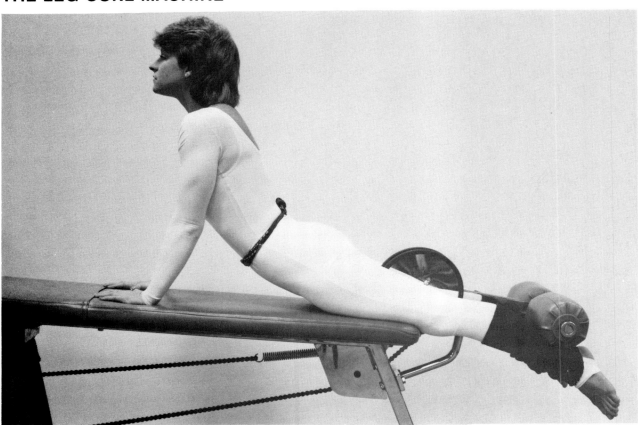

1. Position feet beneath rollers before laying down on pad. Knees should be just off the pad surface.

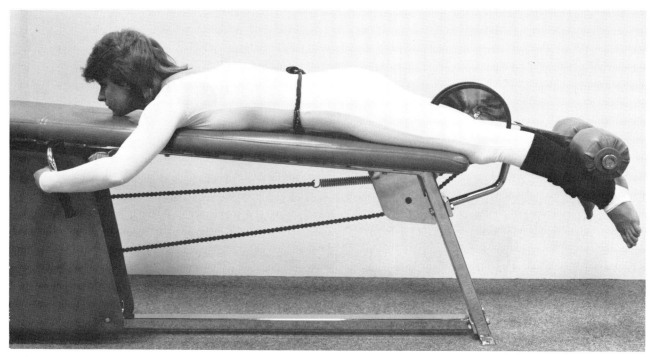

1. Starting position. Feet are flexed slightly downward.

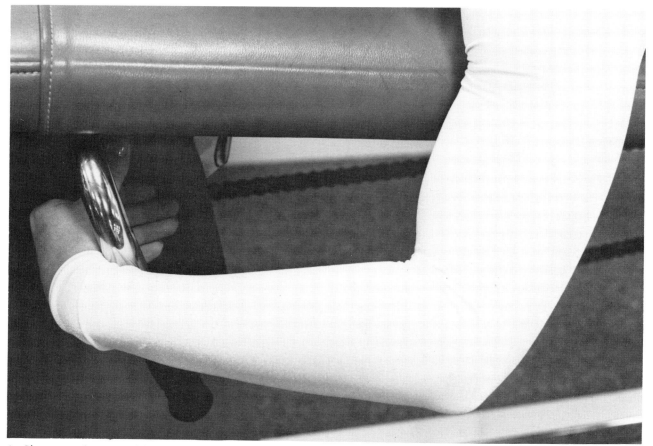

1. Close-up of grip. Holding with flexed wrists prevents you from squeezing hard enough with your handgrip to dangerously raise blood pressure.

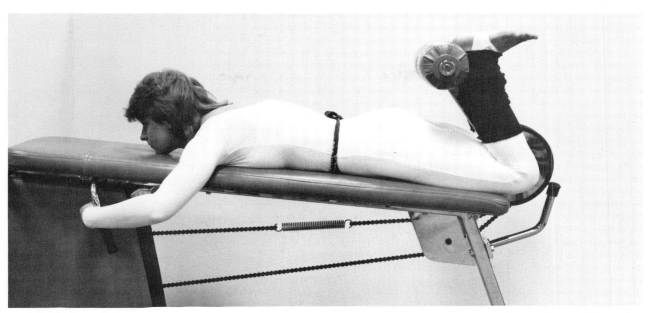

1. Flex slowly upward as far as possible while keeping the hips *down.*
2. *Do not* let your buttocks rise to increase the range of motion. You were simply taught incorrectly if you train that way now. With work you will get the same range of motion, better results, and a healthier back from keeping the hips down.

THE ADDUCTOR MACHINE (AND COMBINATION ADDUCTOR/ABDUCTOR)

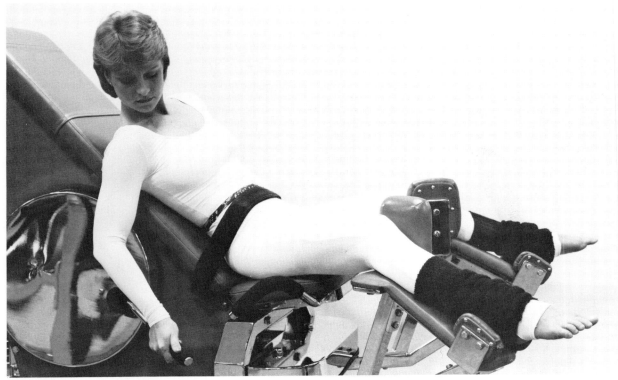

1. Familiarize yourself with the adjustment lever. Pushing it in and turning it counterclockwise will separate the knee pads and increase your range of motion.

2. Through trial and error, set the machine so that your legs are abducted (separated) as widely as possible. The adjustment procedure will be identical on the Combination Ad/Ab machine.

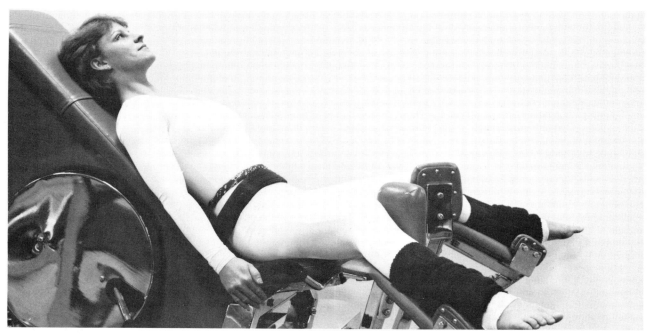

1. With the torso and head back and relaxed, squeeze the legs together. Pressure should be exerted by rolling the knees slightly inward. The feet are along for the ride and do nothing.

2. Squeeze and hold in the fully contracted position for a count of two, then slowly return to the abducted position.

THE ABDUCTOR MACHINE

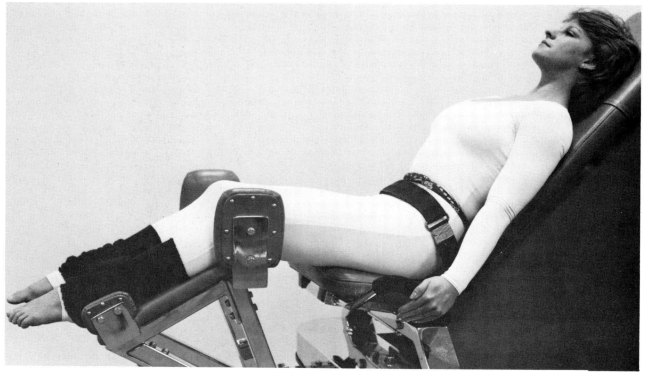

1. Sit back, relax, and belt in. If your knees do not meet the knee pads (short people only, for the most part), use a full-length back pad behind you.

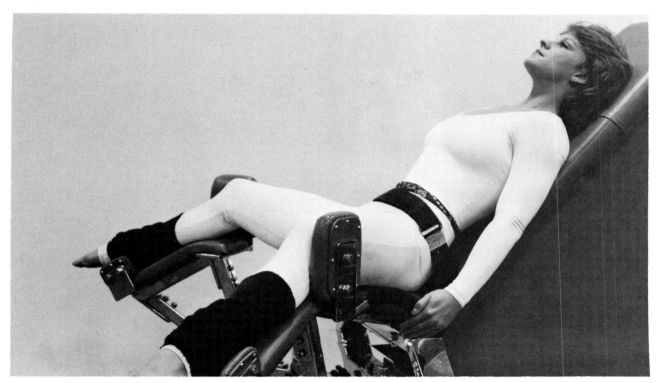

1. Abduct (separate) the legs slowly and as fully as possible. Press with the knees, not the feet.
2. Hold this abducted position for a count of two then return to the adducted starting position.

Touch and go—do not rest the weight stack.
3. If you are on the Combination Ad/Ab machine, simply spin the knee pads so that they are outside the knees, then proceed as above.

THE MULTI-EXERCISE MACHINE CALF RAISE

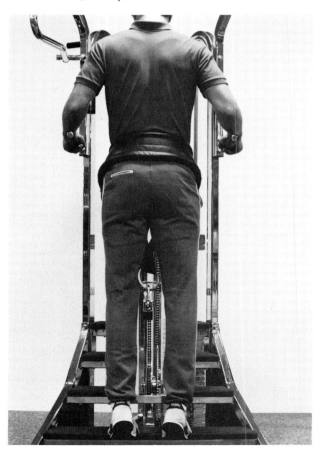

1. Attach the hip belt to the machine's lever.
2. Climb through the belt and position it above your pelvic girdle. It should be in a snug, secure position.
3. Climb to the second step of the platform (new models) or first step (old, adjustable-carriage models).
4. While holding onto the triceps dip bars, raise on your toes as high as possible and hold for a count of two.
5. Lower as fully as possible and repeat.

THE MULTI-EXERCISE MACHINE FOOT FLEXOR

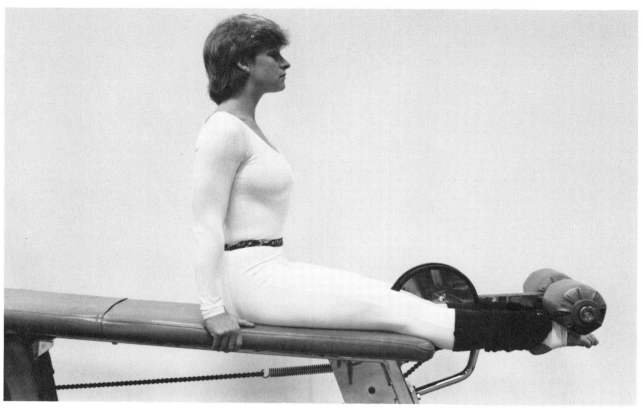

1. Sit erect and place the feet below the rollers. This exercise can be done with (safest) or without footwear.

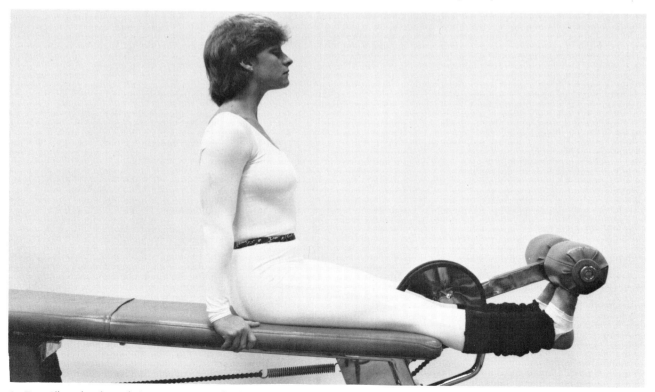

1. Dorsiflex the feet (bring toes towards shins) as fully as possible.
2. Move your body backward or forward until you find the position that allows comfortable and full foot movement.

THE HIP FLEXOR MACHINE

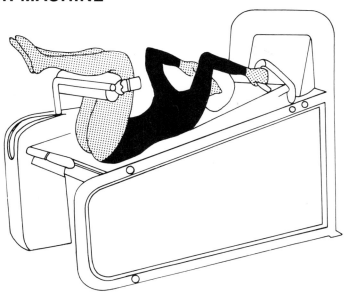

1. Sit and fasten belt across the lower thighs.
2. Lie back and grasp overhead handles with an open grip.

3. Slowly flex your legs toward the torso, pausing for a count of two at full hip flexion. Return slowly and repeat.

8
TORSO/SHOULDERS

Our focus here is on the three major muscles/muscle groups of the upper body.

Latissimus Dorsi/Teres Major. With the torso fixed they bring the arms down (pull-down exercise); with the arms fixed they raise the torso (chin-ups).

Pectoralis Major and Minor. They bring the arms toward the midline of the chest in several ways (arm cross or pectoral flye exercise; bench press/incline press exercise).

Deltoids (anterior or front, middle, and posterior or rear). They elevate the arms either to the front, side, or overhead (the latter with help from the triceps).

You should expect to devote about half your workout time to these major or "prime" movers—about two exercises or machines for each. Their importance to both daily living and athletic success cannot be overestimated.

Muscles	Nautilus® Machines	Muscles	Nautilus® Machines
Latissimus/Teres Major	Pullover, Pullover/Torso Arm, Behind Neck, Behind Neck/Torso Arm, Torso Arm (free-standing), Multi-Exercise Chin-Ups		Overhead Press (freestanding), 70° Shoulder, 40° Chest/Shoulder, Multi-Exercise Upright Rowing (see Chapter 9), Rowing Torso (rear deltoid only)
Pectoralis Major/Minor	Double Chest, Women's Chest, 10° Chest, 40° Chest/Shoulder	Trapezius/Rhomboids	Rowing Torso, Neck and Shoulder
Deltoids	Double Shoulder, Lateral Raise (freestanding),	Neck	Four-Way Neck, Rotary Neck, Neck and Shoulder

Muscles	Nautilus® Machines
Rectus Abdominus	Abdominal Machine
Obliques and Transverse Abdominus	Rotary Torso
Low Back Extensors	Low Back Machine

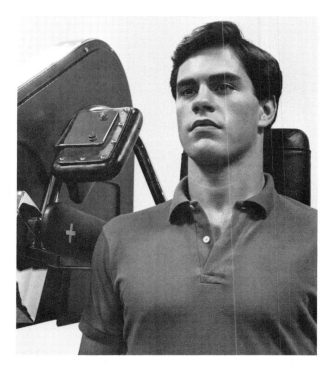

THE PULLOVER MACHINE

Right:

1. Set seat height so that the axis of cam rotation (cross on padding) aligns with the approximate axis of shoulder rotation. This point will be about an inch below the top of your deltoids.

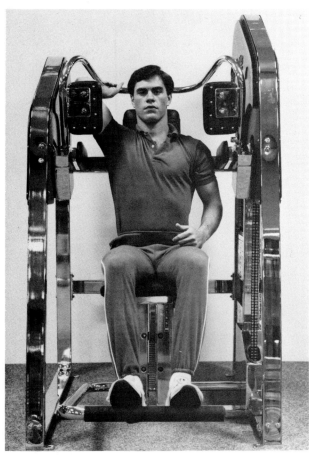

1. Press the foot lever downward to bring the crossbar into position.
2. Grasp the crossbar with one hand to bring it comfortably forward.

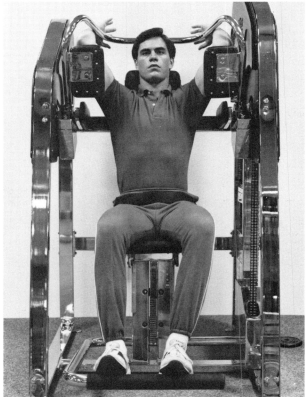

1. Place elbows in the pads and the hands alongside the crossbar. Do not grasp the crossbar with a closed grip.
2. Keep feet on lever until correct position is attained. Sit against back pad and make sure belt is secure.

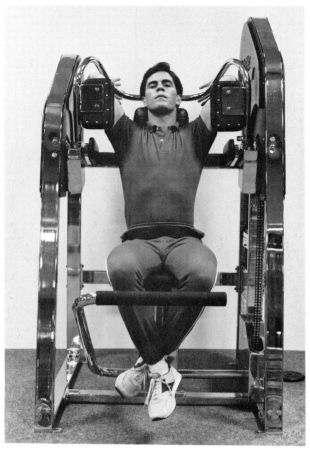

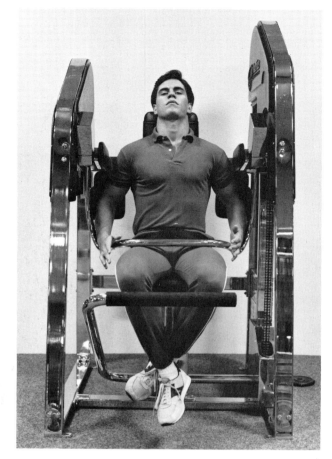

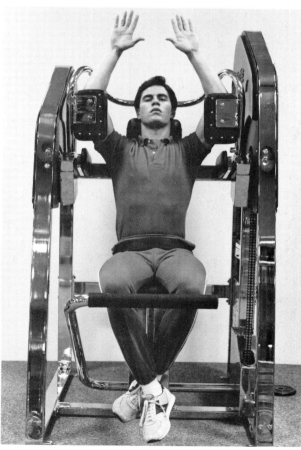

Above, left:
1. Remove feet from the lever.
2. Let machine slowly draw you backward into the stretched position.
3. When first learning the use of the machine, use light weight—you don't want to be forced too far backward by a heavy weight stack. The foot lever can always be used to catch the stack if you're in trouble.

Above, right:
1. Slowly bring the crossbar over and down to your abdomen or thighs.
2. Notice the open grip. The movement is performed *completely* through pressure from the elbows. Do not pull the crossbar with your hands (which would greatly reduce latissimus involvement).
3. Pause for a count of two, then return slowly to a full but completely pain-free stretch.

Below, left:
1. Variation: For even greater latissimus isolation, try using the surface of your upper arms against the elbow pads. This will prevent you quite successfully from using your hands!

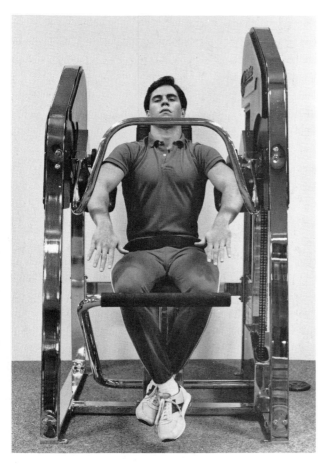

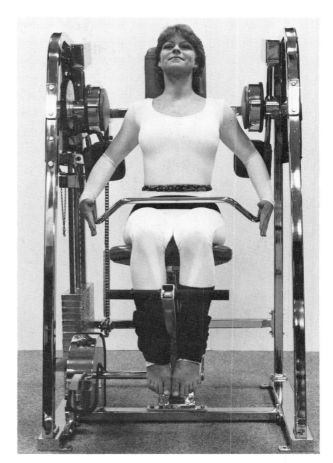

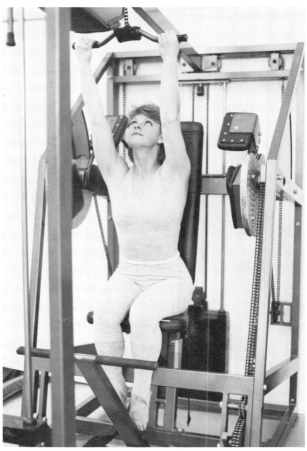

Above, left:

1. Near-finishing position on pullover variation.
2. Get as complete a range of motion as possible, but stay pain-free in the stretched position.

Above, right:

1. The Women's Pullover: Follow the same instructions as for the men's unit.

THE PULLOVER/TORSO ARM MACHINE

1. Following completion of the Pullover exercise, remove seat belt and reach up to grab Torso Arm bar with palms facing your body. If a spotter or trainer is available, stay belted and have him/her hand you the bar.

Right:
1. Pull bar slowly down to chest. Get as full a range of movement as possible.
2. If you cannot fully extend your arms in the starting position, lower the seat as necessary.

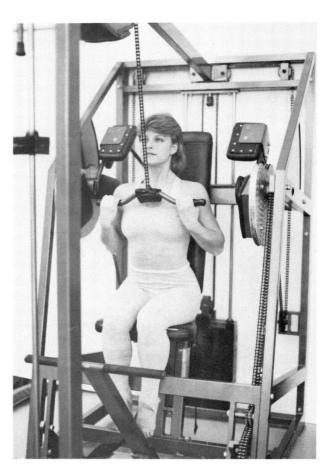

THE BEHIND NECK/TORSO ARM MACHINE

Below, left:
1. Set seat height so that the axis of shoulder rotation (see Pullover) matches the axis of cam rotation.
2. Place arms inside rollers and assume starting position: head is tilted slightly forward to allow arms to cross behind. Palms face directly forward.

Below, right:
1. Squeeze downward while keeping palms facing forward and fingers pointing directly at ceiling.
2. Hold rollers against sides for a count of two then return to starting position and repeat.

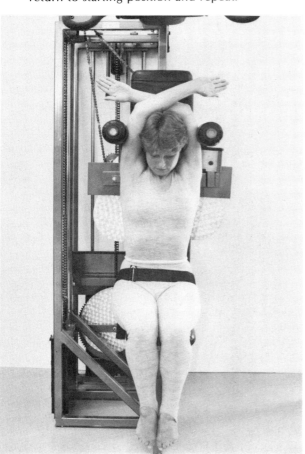

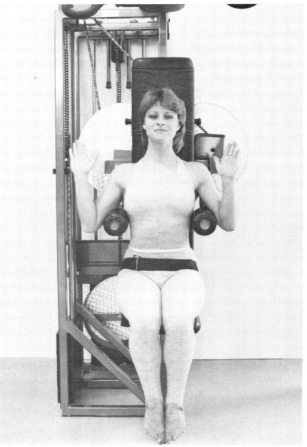

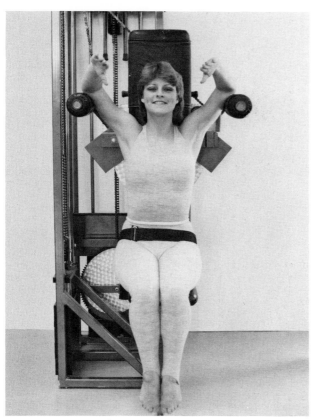

1. For a variation, have arms facing forward and exert pressure with inside of the upper arm/elbow.

1. The Torso Arm Exercise: You may need to remove the seat belt to reach the bar. Shown here is the first of two possible handgrips.

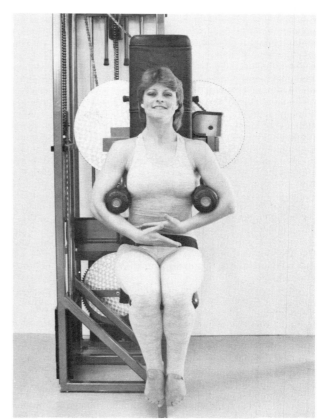

1. Finishing position. Squeeze rollers, hold for two, return and repeat.

1. Lean forward. Bring the bar down to the neck or upper shoulders. Hold for a count of two then return.

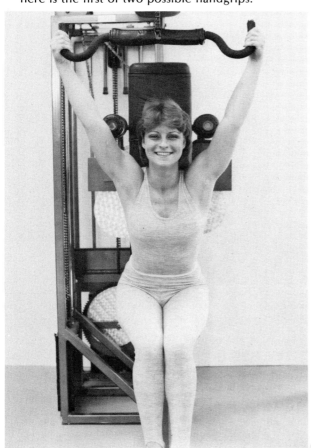

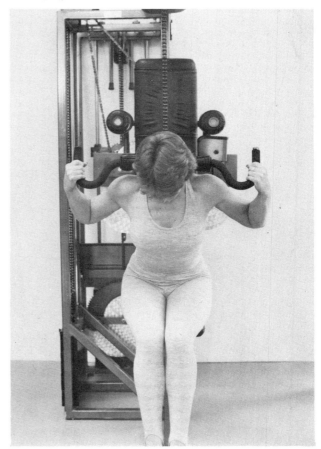

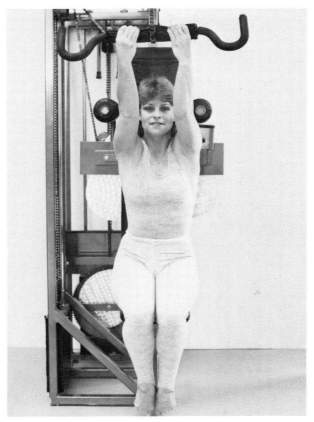

1. Alternate hand grip. This will place slightly greater stress on the elbow flexors (biceps and brachialis).

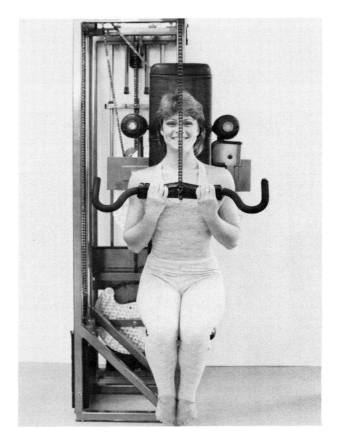

1. You may have to adjust seat height to get the longest possible range of motion. As always, pause for two at full contraction then return slowly and repeat.

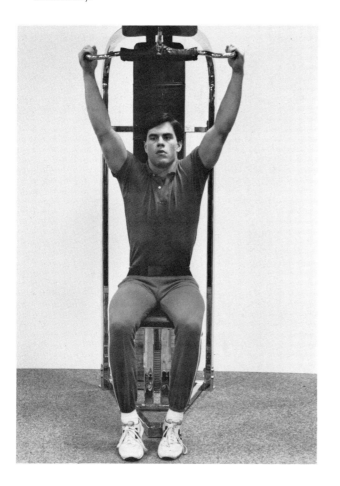

THE TORSO ARM MACHINE

1. Starting position, palms facing inward. Seat height is set so that arms can be fully extended.

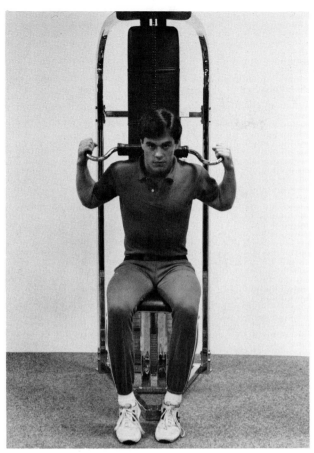

1. Finishing position. Hold bar on neck for a count of two then return slowly and repeat.

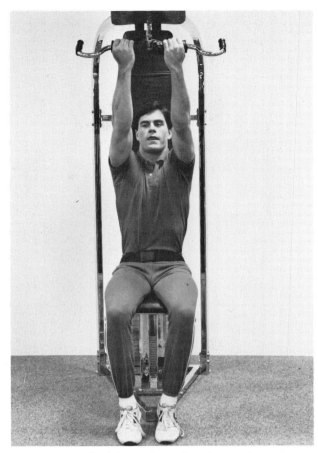

1. Biceps-emphasizing grip. Follow instructions as above.

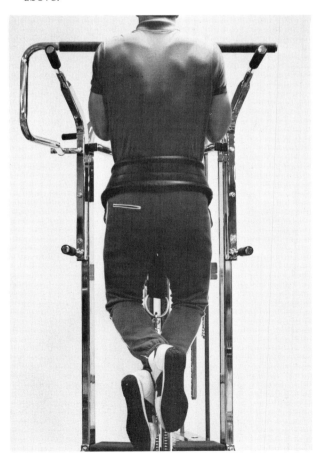

MULTI-EXERCISE MACHINE CHIN-UPS

1. Chins can be done with the hip belt to add to your body weight or without.
2. On older models of the Multi-Exercise, adjust the carriage by lifting the two levers. Your chin should be just above the chinning bar when you climb to the top step.
3. On the new, nonadjustable models, use the appropriate step or pull yourself up into the over-the-bar position.
4. Flex legs and cross ankles.

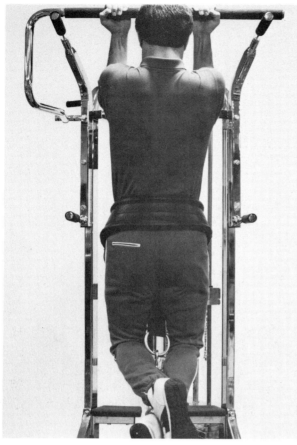

Left:

1. With hands about shoulder width apart, lower yourself slowly into the fully extended position.
2. If you can perform at least five full positive and negative chins (lowering then lifting into starting position), you may use negative-only chins as a bonus. If you cannot do five chins, perform negative-only chins for at least nine workouts.
3. Negative-only: Lower to a count of ten then climb back up steps and repeat. Shoot for at least six negative chins; rest sufficiently between each to make this a more easily-reached goal.

THE DOUBLE CHEST MACHINE

Below, left:

1. The Arm Cross exercise. Seat height is set so that the upper arms form a 90° angle with the torso.
2. Keep head and back relaxed against pad.
3. Pressure is exerted by the forearms. Do not use a closed grip. Keep your thumbs hooked underneath the grips and your fingers back.
4. Get a full stretch in the starting position.

Below, right:

1. Midposition. Note the 90° angles between upper and lower arms and upper arm and torso, and the open grips.

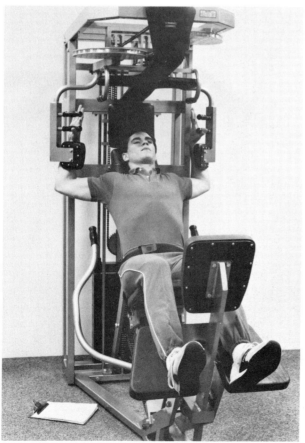

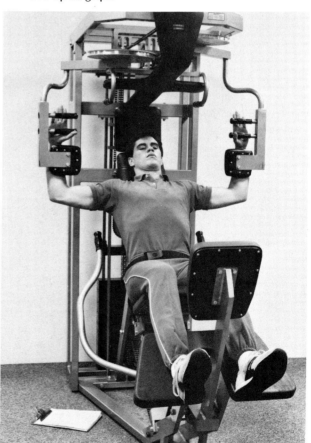

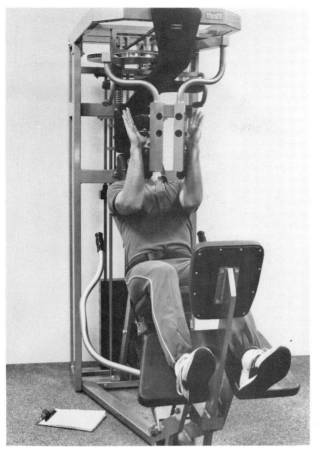

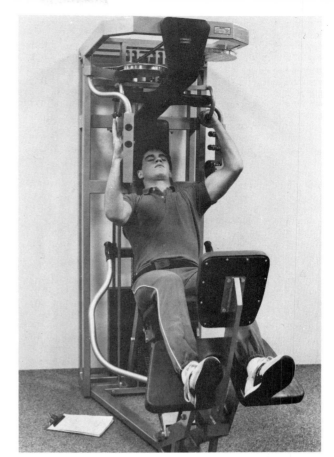

1. Finishing position. Pressure is still being exerted by the forearms. Elbows are directly below the hands. Do not let the elbows flare out to the sides—this reduces pectoralis isolation.
2. Squeeze and hold for a count of two then return to the fully stretched, starting position.

1. One-arm variation. Grasp overhead grip with one hand then follow instructions as above with other arm.

1. The Incline Press exercise. (For unknown reasons, Nautilus has been calling this a decline press for years. Since the head sure looks to me like it's *higher* than the feet, this is an *incline* press. Sorry, Nautilus.) Bring levers into position by pressing out with the feet.
2. Palms may face each other or grasp from above (see next photo).

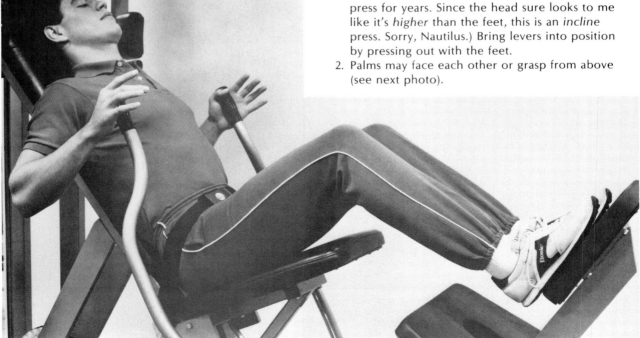

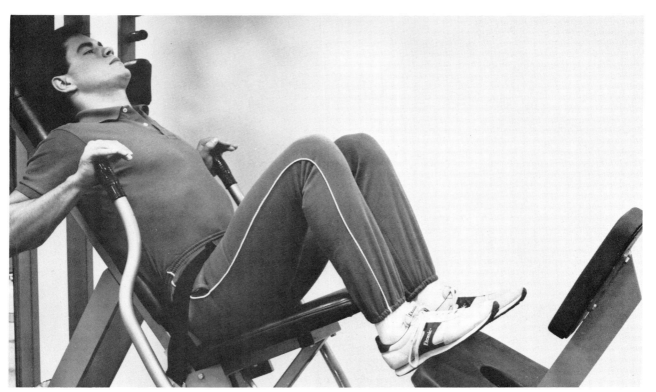

1. Hands are in typical barbell grip position, but not tightly closed around handles. This is starting position.

2. Feet may be rested in this manner to take stress off the lower back. (Try this with the Arm Cross exercise as well.)

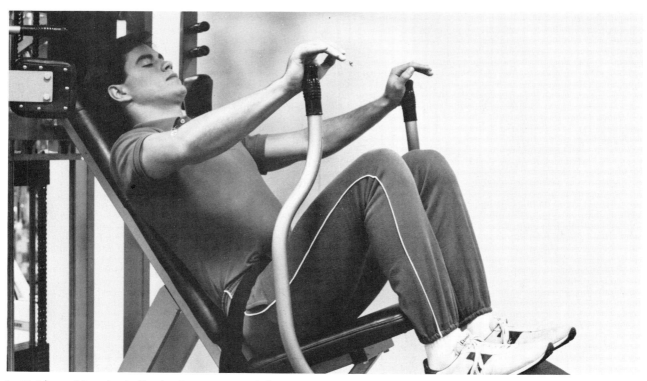

1. Finish position, barbell grip. Do not go to full extension, where you can (a) rest by locking out and (b) damage your elbow joint by moving too quickly.

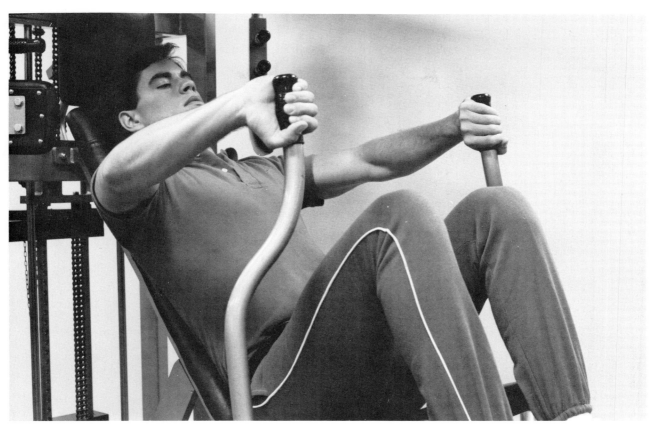

1. Reverse grip position. Use less weight! This is also a great forearm exercise.

1. For negative-emphasized exercise, a trainer may add to the weight stack's downward pull by squatting up against the foot pedal. This is obviously an advanced variation, and must be done carefully.

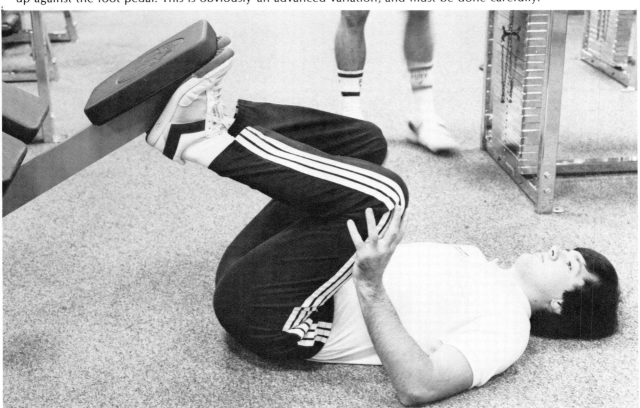

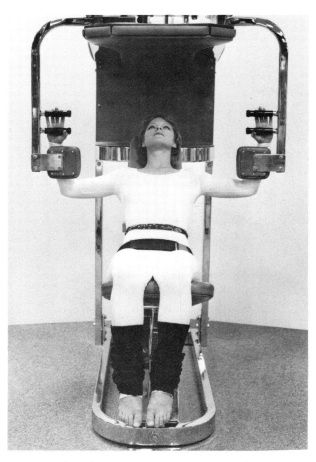

Left:
1. The Women's Chest Machine. Follow instructions as for the Arm Cross exercise.

THE DOUBLE SHOULDER MACHINE

Below, left:
1. The Lateral Raise. Set seat height so the axis of shoulder rotation (see Pullover) matches the axis of cam rotation.
2. Keep an open grip and lead with the elbows.

Below, right:
1. Finishing position. Go no higher than a 90° angle between upper arm and torso. Lower arms are parallel to the floor.
2. Keep head and shoulders back and relaxed. Do not let your shoulders "hunch up" or shrug during the exercise.

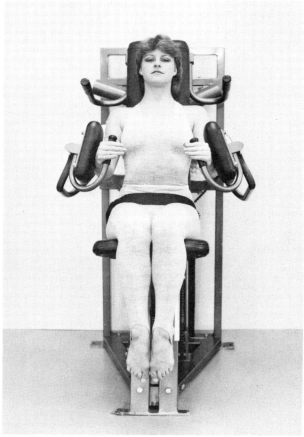

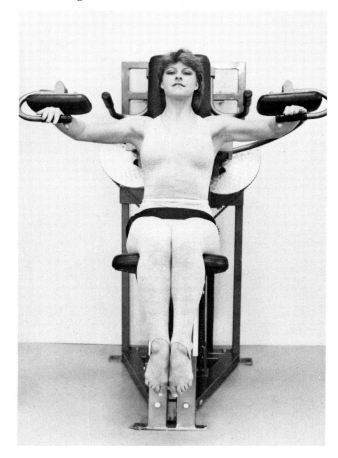

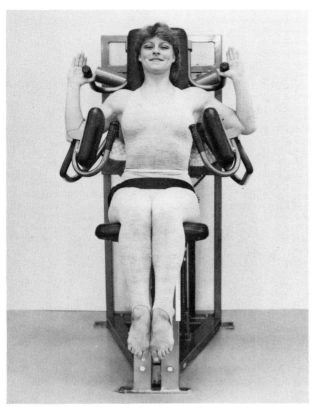

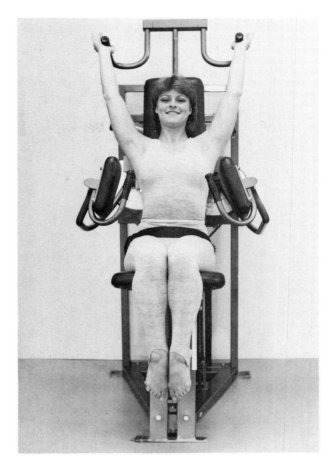

1. The Overhead Press. Again note the open grip. If the seat is raised you will get a longer range of motion, so don't be afraid to unbelt and climb out of the machine briefly.

1. Many people find the standard overhead press position painful to the shoulder. Turning and facing the back pad seems to reduce stress and eliminate the problem.

1. Finishing position. Extend the arms to just short of the lock out position.

1. Finishing position. Note open grip and arms just short of lock out.

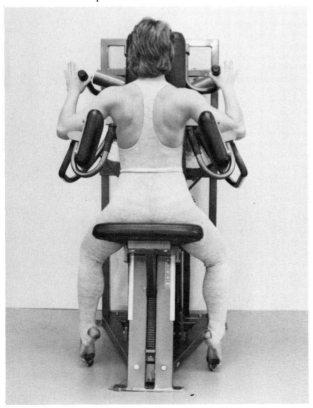

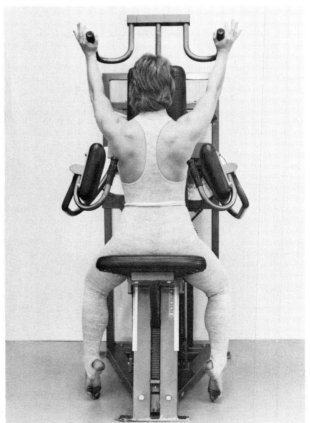

LATERAL RAISE MACHINE

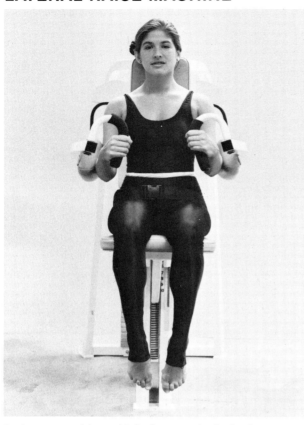

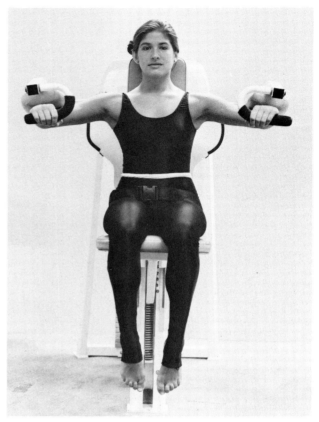

1. A new machine which does not include the overhead press. Redesign of the arm pads has improved on the original model. Instructions for use, however, are identical.

1. Finishing position.

70° SHOULDER MACHINE

1. Set seat height so that the head rests fully on its pad.
2. Place arms under rollers and face palms forward.

1. Bring arms overhead, pause for two, return. Palms still facing outward.

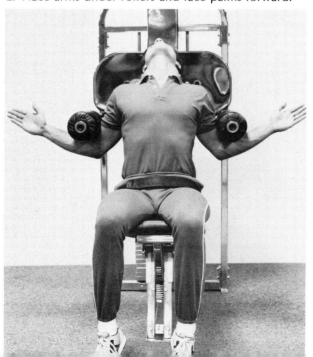

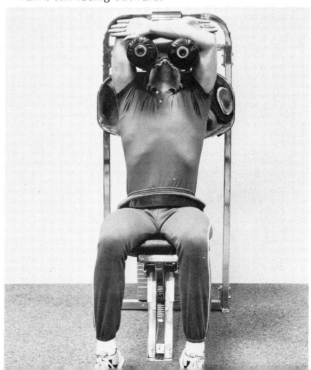

40° CHEST/SHOULDER MACHINE

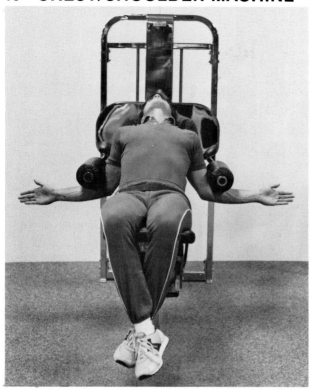

1. Follow instructions as on 70° Shoulder machine.

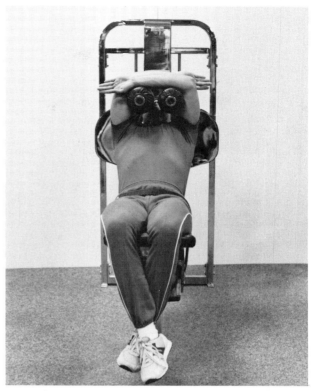

1. Finishing position.

10° CHEST MACHINE

1. Position body so that the upper arms form a 70°–90° angle with the torso. Palms face forward.

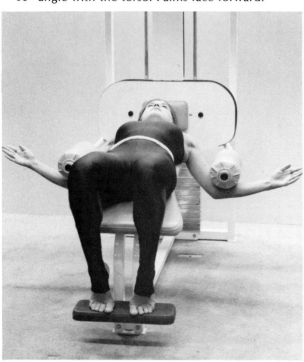

1. Contract then pause for a count of two overhead. Return and repeat.

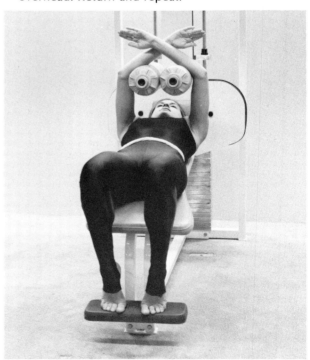

THE ROWING TORSO MACHINE

Right:
1. Sit against the front pad and place arms in front of rollers at a 90° angle to torso.

Below, left:
1. Slowly push backward as far as is comfortable. Hold in this position for a count of two then return slowly to starting position and repeat.
2. Remaining pressed into the front pad will help prevent you from arching your back as you contract.

Below, right:
1. Alternate arm placement that reduces stress on the shoulder joint. Starting position shown here.

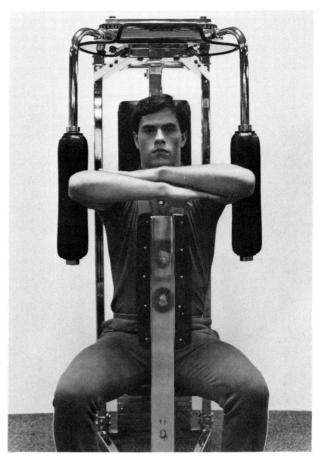

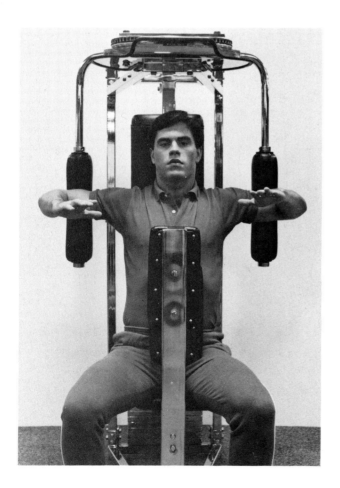

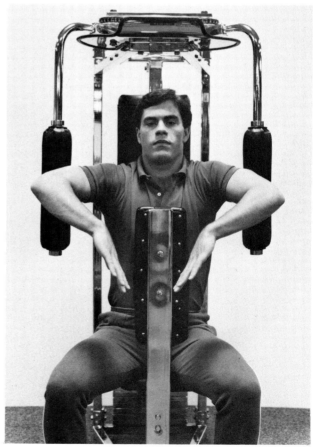

Right:

1. Finishing position for reduced shoulder-stress variation.

THE FOUR-WAY NECK MACHINE

Below, left:

1. Anterior (front) Flexion. Set seat height so that your head makes full contact with the face pads.
2. Sit upright, grasp the crossbar with one hand and one handgrip with the other.
3. Let the head slowly extend backward by gradually reducing the assistance of the hand and assuming the load with the front neck muscles (in a negative or eccentric contraction). Place the second hand on the remaining handgrip.

Below, right:

1. From the fully extended position (head back), bring the head forward while keeping the torso completely motionless.
2. Pause in the contracted position then return slowly toward extension and repeat.

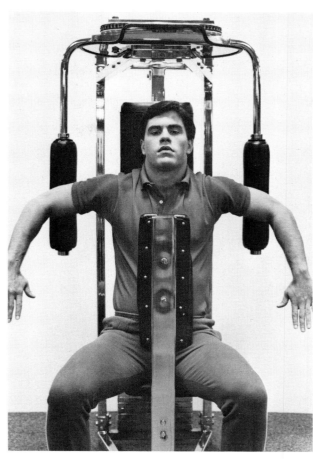

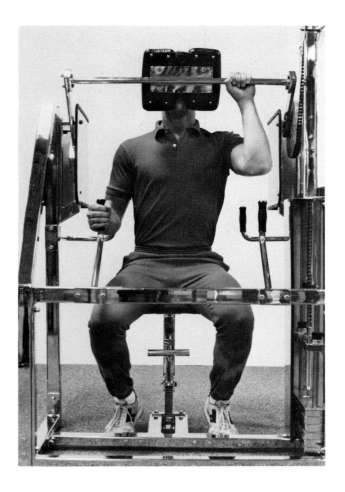

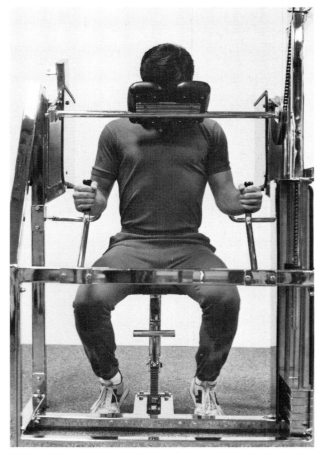

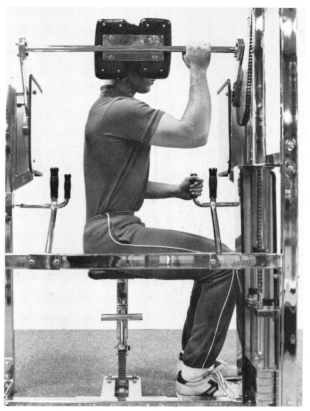

1. Lateral Flexion to the Right. Turn the body 90°
   and follow instructions as for front flexion.

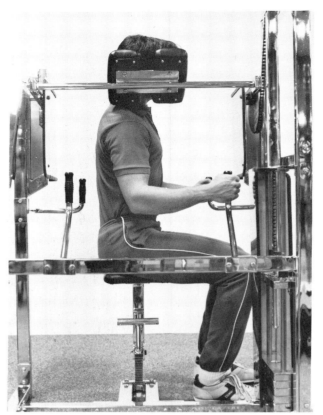

1. The torso again remains completely motionless
   and upright while the head flexes from side to side.
2. Turn 180° and work lateral flexion to the left.

1. Posterior (rear) Flexion. Follow instructions as for
   photo above right.

1. Keep the torso steady and the back straight while
   flexing and extending the head.

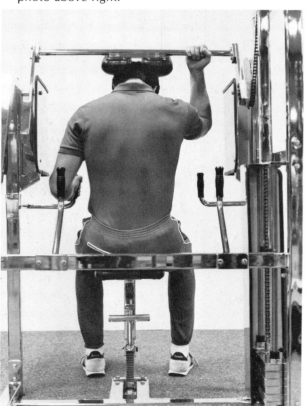

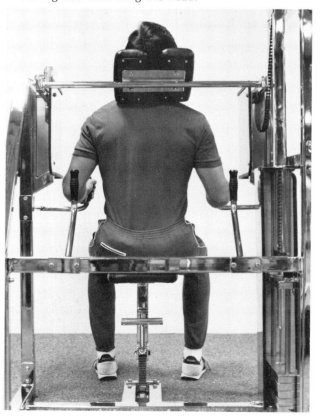

THE ROTARY NECK MACHINE

1. Get familiar with the lever that adjusts the head pads. You'll need to create a snug fit around your head to use this machine properly.
2. When you push the long, right-hand lever (to your side, that is) or pull the left lever, the head will be forced to rotate to the left. Your goal is to resist your arms (no weight stack here!) with the muscles that rotate the neck. Pushing the right-hand lever will therefore enable negative-only training of the neck rotator muscles that prevent rotation to the left.
3. Get familiar with the action of the two long levers before beginning a set.
4. Work one complete rotation from right to left and resist with your neck rotators.
5. Reverse your arm action and resist left-to-right rotation with your neck.
6. Do only six repetitions to each side.
7. Do not use this machine if you have a history of neck or upper back problems.

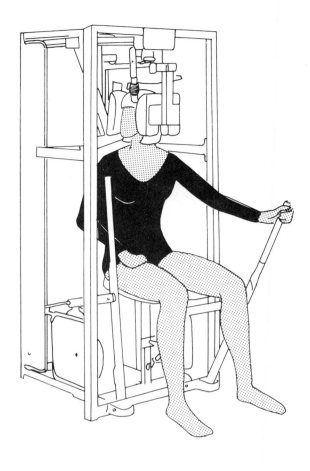

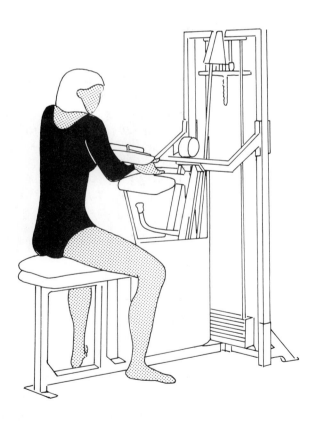

THE NECK AND SHOULDER MACHINE

1. You are in the correct starting position when the weight load you have chosen is elevated off the weight stack with your shoulders down and relaxed. Most people will need to sit atop two or more pads to bring them to this starting height.
2. Arms are threaded between the forearm pads with palms facing up.
3. In the relaxed, shoulders-down position, remember that the weight stack you've chosen should be elevated.
4. Shrug your shoulders as high as possible, lifting the weight with the trapezius muscles and not the biceps. You may want to practice shoulder shrugs outside the machine first.
5. Hold in the elevated position for a count of two then return slowly and repeat.

THE ABDOMINAL MACHINE

Below, left:
1. Set seat height so that the tip of your sternum matches the indicated point on the machine.

Right:
1. Forget about the handgrips—the ones that should never have been put there in the first place. Help isolate your abdominals by threading your lower arms up and through the handles. This will reduce your ability to pull with your arms. (By the way, Nautilus corrected their error here and is now introducing an Abdominal Machine that places resistance against the torso—the way it should have been done the first time.)
2. Forget about the pad on the seat that tells you how widely to separate your legs. It's not too swift either. The wider you can spread your legs, the less the hip flexors can help your abdominals. This is an *abdominal* machine, not a hip flexor/upper body machine!

Below, right:
1. Contract with your abdominals *only*. This is an extremely difficult machine when done correctly, even with only one plate. If you cannot create enough force with your abdominals alone, add some assistance from the legs, arms, or both.
2. Do not contract through the full range of the machine's motion (another design mistake). Your rectus abdominus only works through one-third to one-half the range of machine travel. After that you must bring in the hip flexors and torso. Go halfway, hold for two, then return. Touch and go with the weight stack.

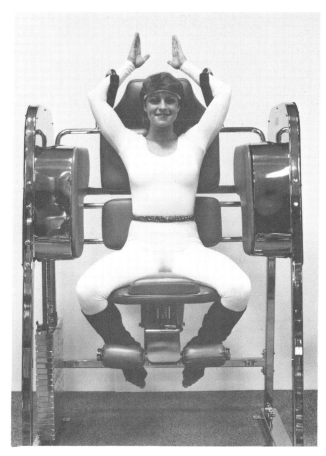

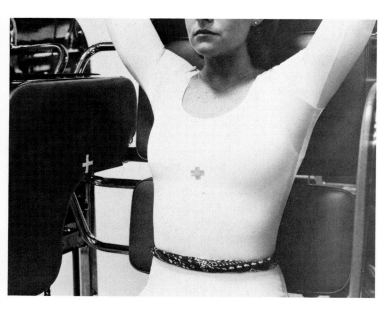

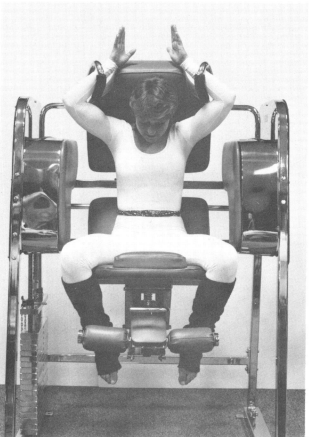

THE ROTARY TORSO MACHINE

Right:

1. Sit upright and cross arms, gripping with the thumbs only. Begin by facing straight ahead. Your nose should be centered between the two vertical bars, and should *never* leave this position.

Below, left:

1. Relax and rotate away from the weight stack into the stretched, starting position. Do not let your gaze stray from between the two bars.

Below, right:

1. Contract and rotate toward the stack. Keep your back as straight as possible and your gaze fixed. This is *not* an arm exercise, so don't use any muscles but your obliques (and transverse abdominus).
2. Do a full set of reps on one side then turn and repeat for the other.

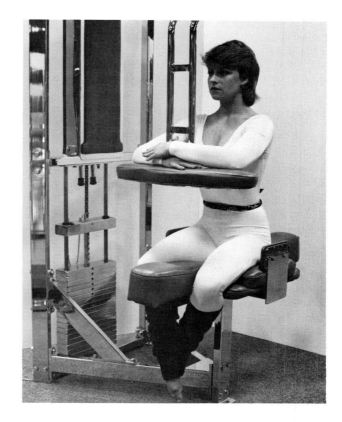

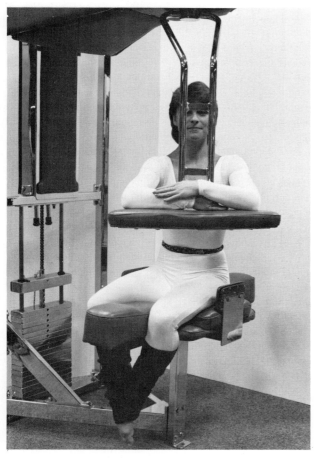

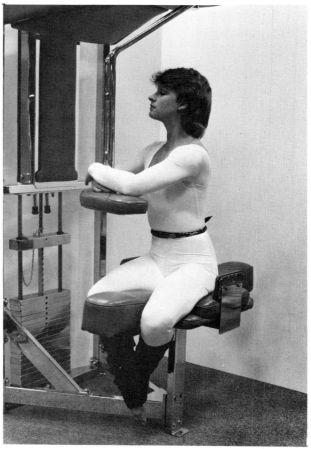

THE LOWER BACK MACHINE

THIS MACHINE SHOULD ABSOLUTELY NOT BE USED BY ANYONE WITH BACK PAIN, A PAST HISTORY OF BACK PAIN, OR NUMBNESS/TINGLING SENSATIONS IN THE LOWER BODY *WITHOUT* EXPRESS MEDICAL, CHIROPRACTIC, OR OSTEOPATHIC PERMISSION. IT IS A POTENTIALLY DANGEROUS MACHINE, AND SHOULD BE USED ONLY IF YOU HAVE A COMPLETELY SYMPTOM-FREE BACK (OR HAVE BEEN CLEARED). MANY BACK CONDITIONS CAN BE WORSENED BY USE OF THIS MACHINE.

Below, left:
1. Place one leg over the seat and straddle the machine.

Below, right:
1. Sit and find a comfortable and stable position for your feet. Rotate the large thigh pads and try placing your feet either on the step or on the base.

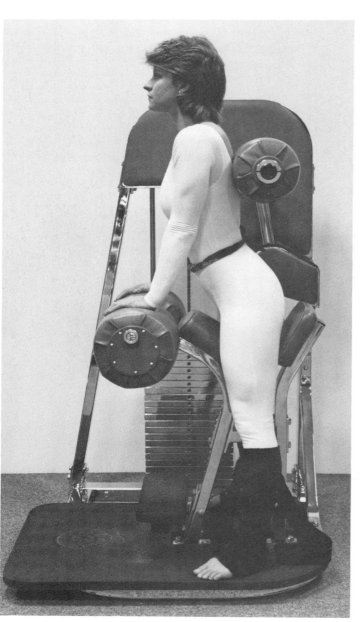

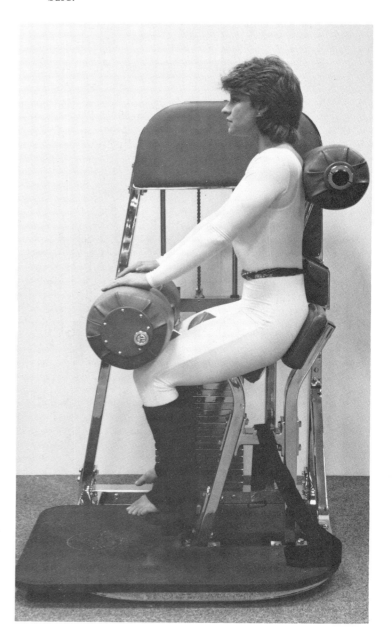

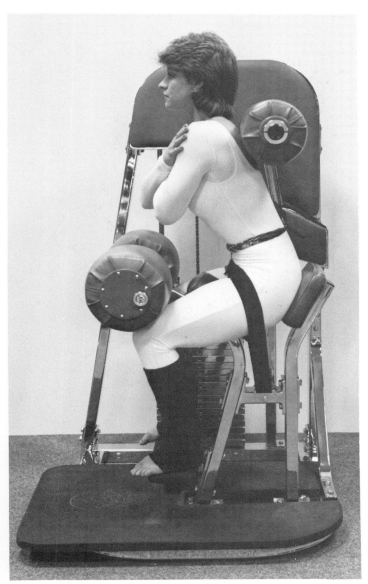

1. Belt in, cross arms, and lean forward slowly until the weight stack touches down.

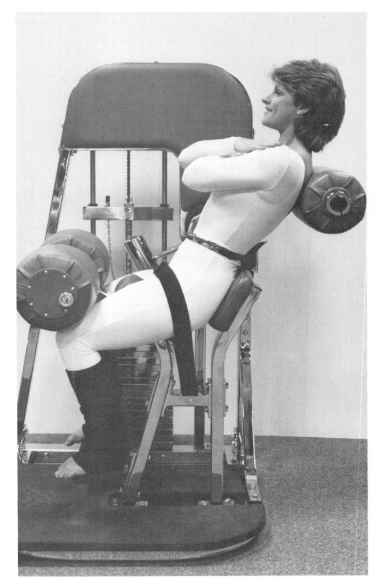

1. Contract and lean back slowly, going no further than a flat back position. Do not hyperextend the back. Hold for a count of two then return and repeat.

9
THE ARMS

Your workout is winding down; only the arms remain. The Multi-Biceps and -Triceps units offer a host of variations, and the accurately-named Multi-Exercise machine comes in quite handy as well.

Beginners should start with the simple bilateral curls (both arms working together). Next in the progression is unilateral training, where one arm either relaxes while the other completes a full rep, or holds isometrically in the *contracted* position while the other does a full rep. (These apply to the Multi-Triceps as well.) Other variations include: one-arm curls; one-arm, negative-only curls; isometrics; and infimetrics/akinetics. More on these variations follow.

Muscle Groups	Nautilus® Machines	Muscle Groups	Nautilus® Machines
Elbow Flexors			Exercise Triceps Extension, Multi-Exercise Dips, Overhead Press, Incline Press, Pullover
Brachialis, Biceps Brachii	Multi-Biceps, Plateloading Biceps, Multi-Exercise Biceps Curls, Torso Arm, Multi-Exercise Chin-Ups, Multi-Exercise Upright Rowing		
		Wrist Flexors	
		Flexor Carpi Radialis and Ulnaris	Multi-Exercise Wrist Curls
Elbow Extensors			
Three heads of Triceps Brachii	Multi-Triceps, Plateloading Triceps, Multi-	*Wrist Extensors*	
		Extensor Carpi Radialis and Ulnaris	Multi-Exercise Reverse Wrist Curls

80

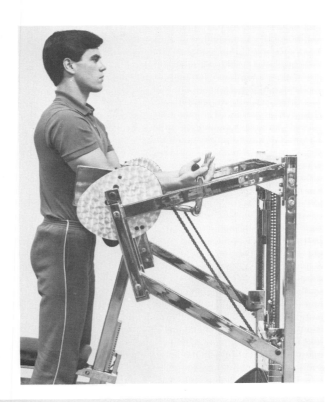

THE MULTI-BICEPS MACHINE

Left:

1. Grasp the handles before sitting down in machine. Note open hand grip.

Middle, left:

1. Set seat height so that a straight line drawn from the shoulder to the hands forms a 15°–20° angle with the floor. This is starting position. Shoulders are down (not shrugged), grip remains open.

Below, left:

1. Both hands may be curled up to full flexion simultaneously (Curl #1, not shown), or one arm may remain extended while the other does a full rep (flexion then extension; Curl #2, shown).
2. For Curl #3, hold the flexed arm isometrically at the ear and do a complete rep with the other arm (extend then flex back to ear; same photo!).
3. Negative-only (Curl #4, not shown): Stand in machine, use two hands on one lever to bring it into the fully flexed position. Sit, then lower to a count of ten with one arm only. Repeat up to ten times, then switch to other arm.

Below, right:

1. Infimetric/Akinetic (Curls #5 and #6): Swing the infimetric bar into place above the weight stack (shown).
2. Pull on both levers simultaneously to bring the top plate (infimetric) or weight stack chosen (akinetic) up against the infimetric bar.
3. Begin curling one arm while resisting with the opposite arm. You will be doing a "concentric" or positive curl with the flexing arm and an "eccentric" or negative curl with the extending arm.
4. Keep the weights against the infimetric bar, taking five to ten seconds to complete one full

(Continued on next page)

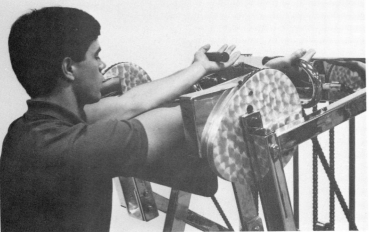

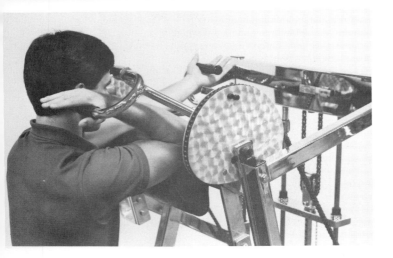

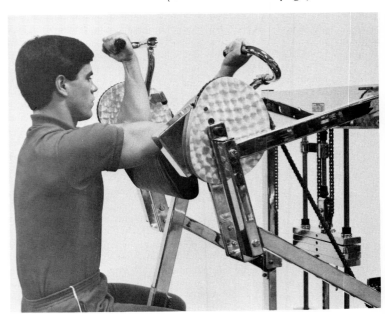

(Continue from previous page)
curl with the flexing arm. Do not release tension
and let the plate(s) drop off the infimetric bar.

5. Shoot for 10–12 curls with each arm.
6. For Curl #7: Isometric exercise can be performed
   with the infimetric bar in place. Since the arm
   that is extending eccentrically can create 30%–
   40% more force than the curling arm, it can
   prevent the curling arm from moving—hence an
   isometric contraction.
7. Begin with the right arm near full extension.
   Attempt to curl the right arm but hold it
   motionless with the eccentric contraction of the
   left arm. Hold a maximal contraction for about
   six seconds.
8. Move about one-third way through the curl then
   do another six-second isometric. Finish the
   exercise near full flexion, then repeat with left
   arm.

THE PLATELOADING BICEPS CURL

Below, left:
1. Sit upright, grasp rotating handlebar in the
   middle with the palms turned slightly inward.
2. Align elbow joint axis with the machine's axis of
   rotation.
3. Keep the shoulders down and relaxed (not
   shrugged).

Above, right:
1. Curl slowly upward, using either a loose, closed
   grip or an open grip. Note good seated posture.

Below, right:
1. Finishing position. Elbows have maintained
   alignment with machine axis; posture is still
   good.

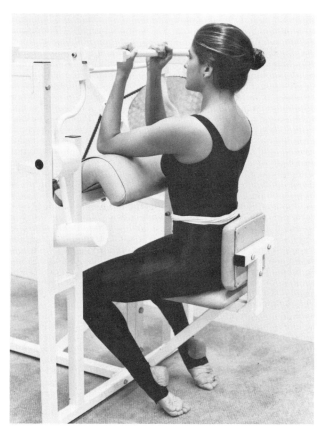

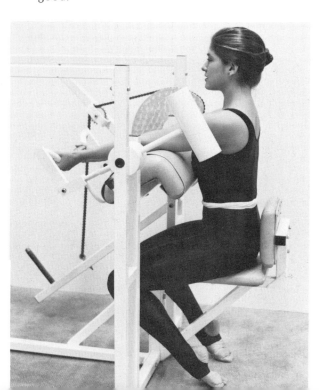

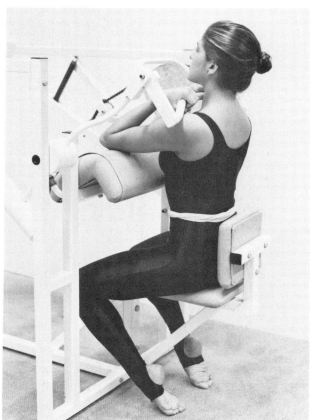

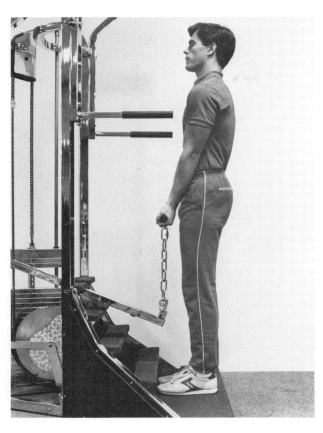

MULTI-EXERCISE MACHINE CURLS

Left:

1. Your range of motion won't be as complete on this machine, so use this exercise only when there's a long line to get to the Multi-Biceps or Plateloader.
2. Starting position. Good posture, elbows at side.

Below, left:

1. Finishing position. Greater range of motion can be obtained by letting the elbows swing slightly forward.
2. Hold in contracted position for a count of two, lower slowly, and repeat.

MULTI-EXERCISE MACHINE UPRIGHT ROWING

1. Same starting posture as left photo but reverse grip.

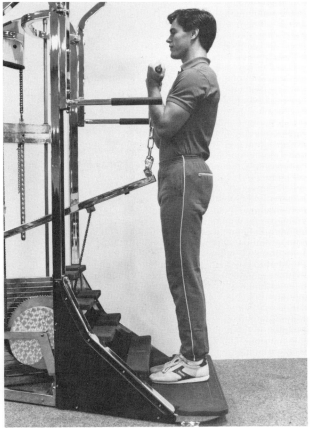

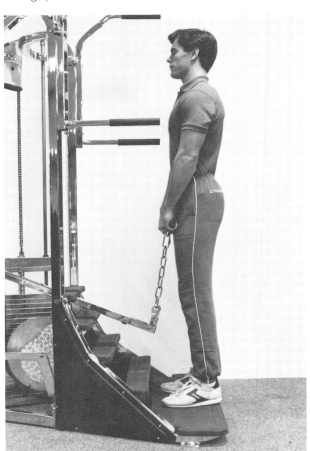

Right:

1. Pull upward slowly to chin, leading with elbows. Note flat back position.
2. Pause for two, lower slowly, and repeat.

THE MULTI-TRICEPS MACHINE

Below, left:

1. Enter machine by straddling seat and pushing levers toward weight stack.

Below, right:

1. Extend both arms. Set seat height so that the straight line from shoulder to hand forms a 15°–20° angle with the floor.

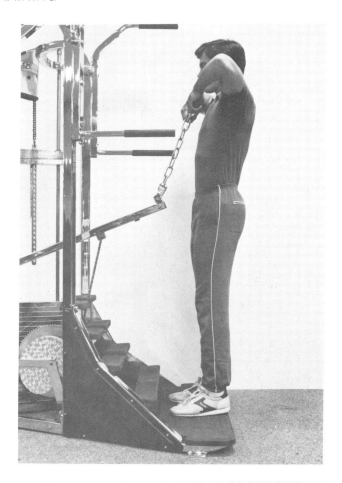

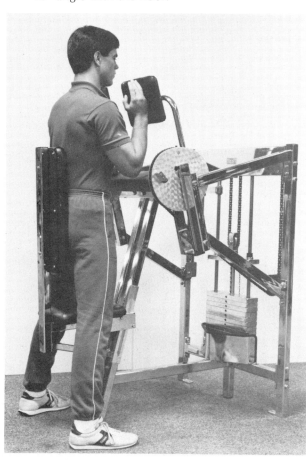

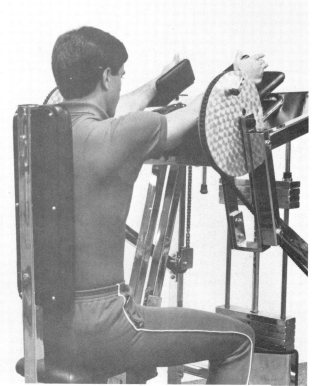

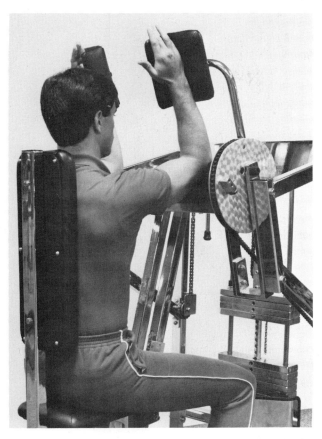

Left:

1. Triceps Extension #1: Let both arms flex and extend simultaneously. Note hands in a "karate chop" position. Elbows are aligned with the center of machine rotation.

Below, left:

1. Triceps Extension #2: Hold one arm isometrically at the relaxed or flexed position and do a complete rep with the other arm (shown). Keep the shoulders down and relaxed.
2. Triceps Extension #3: Hold one arm isometrically in the extended (contracted) position, then do a complete rep with the other arm (same photo).

Below, right:

1. Infimetric/Akinetic (variations #4 and #5): Swing the infimetric bar into place above the weight stack.
2. Follow instructions as for the Multi-Biceps. One arm extends while the other resists. Do not let the top plate (infimetric) or plates (akinetic) drop off the infimetric bar.
3. Take 5–10 seconds to complete one flexion/extension; aim for 10–12 reps with each arm.
4. Isometric Extensions (variation #6): Follow instructions as for Multi-Biceps.

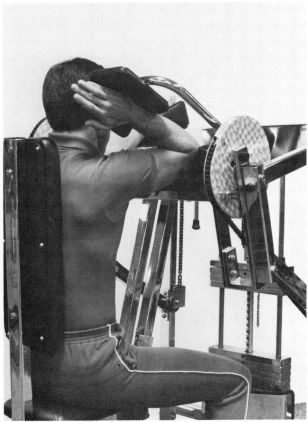

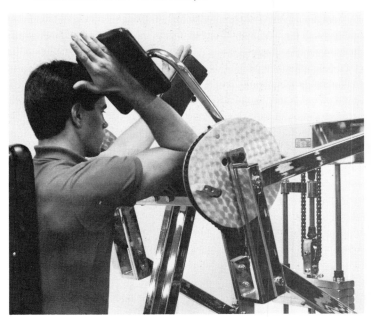

THE PLATELOADING TRICEPS MACHINE

Right:

1. Straddle seat and enter as with Multi-Triceps. The shoulder to hand line should again form a 15°–20° angle with the floor. Use seat pads if the angle is much beyond 20°.
2. Let the machine draw you back into the flexed position.

Below, left:

1. Extend both arms simultaneously. Pause for two, return slowly, and repeat.
2. There is no correlation between the amount of weight you use on the Plateloader and the number of plates on the Multi-Triceps. You'll need to use trial and error to find your correct weight here.

THE MULTI-EXERCISE MACHINE TRICEPS EXTENSION

Below, right:

1. Find a sturdy chair and a long towel. Place chair against base of machine; run towel around chain and bar as shown.
2. Grasp securely with one hand on each end of the towel. Keep your back firmly planted in the chair. Position your arms so that the upper arms run alongside the ears.

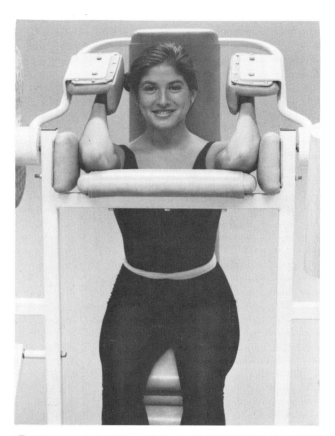

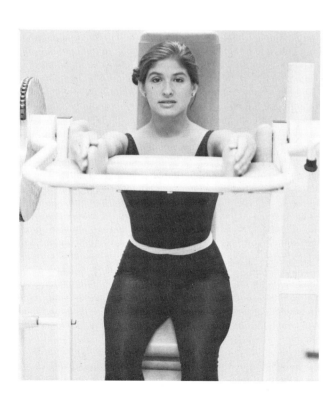

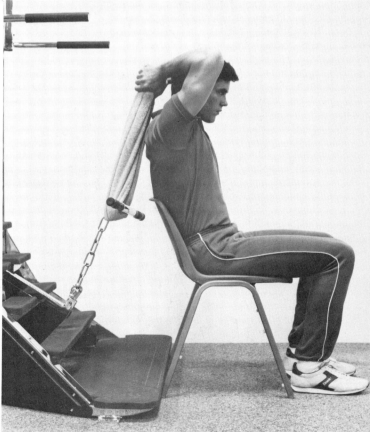

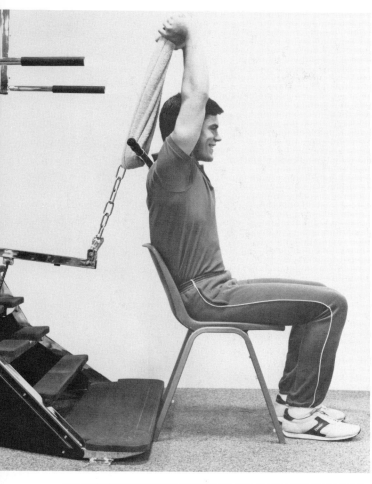

Left:
1. Extend upward slowly keeping the elbows locked against the ears.
2. Hold in contracted position for a count of two, return slowly, and repeat.

MULTI-EXERCISE MACHINE TRICEPS DIPS

Below, left:
1. Starting position. The hip belt may be worn to increase difficulty if your body weight doesn't provide a sufficient challenge to your triceps.
2. On the older, adjustable-carriage Multi-Exercise machines, set the height of the carriage so that you are in the shown starting position when you climb to the top step.
3. If you cannot reach this position on the newer, nonadjustable machines, climb as high as you can, then press up into position.
4. Flex knees and cross ankles.

Below, right:
1. Lower slowly to the point where upper and lower arms form a 90° angle.
2. Press back up into starting position.
3. If you cannot do five complete dips, or wish to use negative-only dips for variety, lower yourself to a count of ten then climb back up the steps and repeat. Shoot for ten negative-only reps, resting sufficiently between each to make this possible.

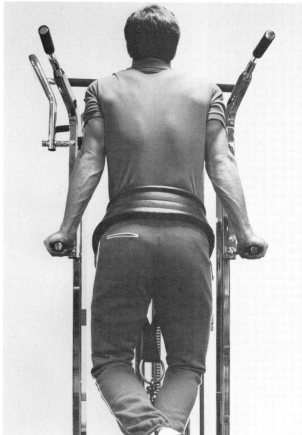

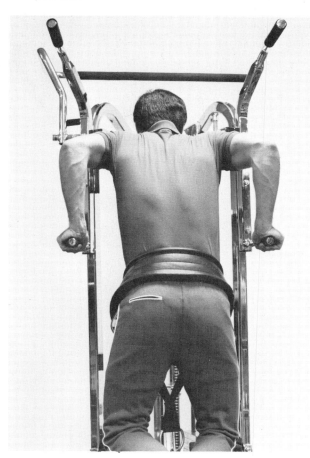

MULTI-EXERCISE MACHINE WRIST CURLS

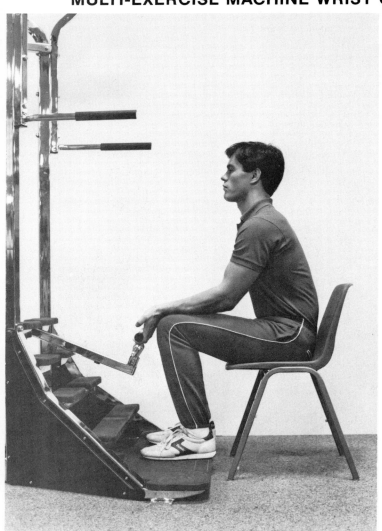 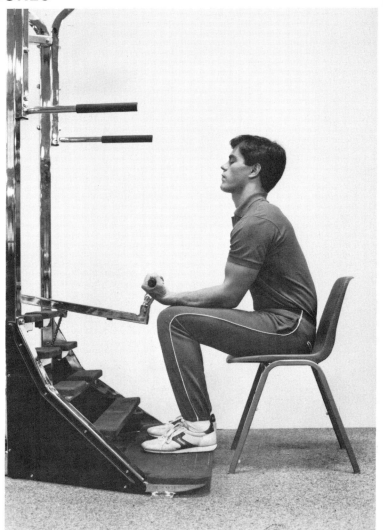

1. Position seat so that when bar is grasped, the hands *only* extend over the knees.
2. Start with the bar held by the fingers only. Keep your back as straight as possible, though some forward lean is required.

1. Begin by curling bar up with fingers.
2. Complete rep by closing grip and flexing hands as far as possible toward the forearms.
3. Pause for a count of two, lower slowly, and repeat.

MULTI-EXERCISE MACHINE REVERSE WRIST CURLS

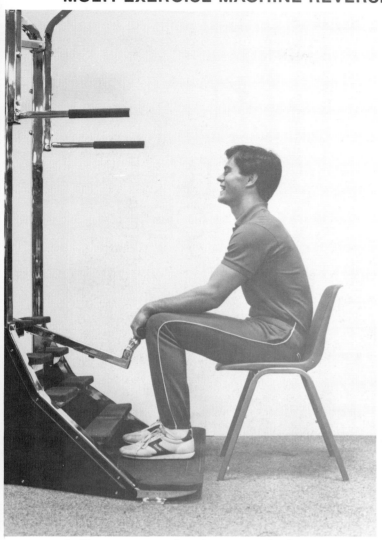 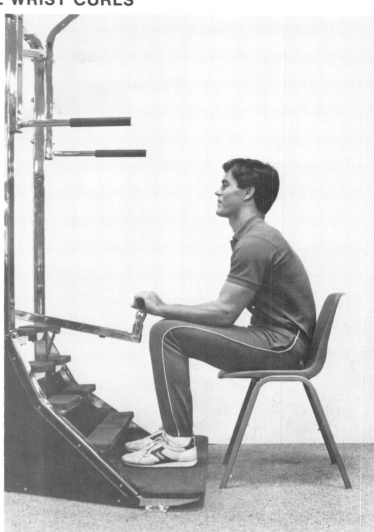

1. Use a reverse, palms-down grip. The fingers must obviously be closed in this exercise.

1. Curl upward as high as possible. Pause for two, lower slowly, and repeat.

10
NAUTILUS WORKOUTS—
BEGINNER TO ADVANCED

Ladies and gentlemen, masochists of all ages: here are enough Nautilus workouts to keep you busy until the Social Security checks start arriving.

Whether you're new to Nautilus or an old hand, remember that *variety* is the key to long-term results. You should spend no more than six weeks on any one workout! Scientists have recently proven that staleness and plateaus set in quickly (a matter of weeks) if machines and exercises aren't varied.

Each time you change workouts expect to spend some time finding the new, correct weights. Don't be in a great rush—by changing exercises you'll be nearly guaranteeing a steadier flow of strength and size improvements. If you find, at any point, that you're plateauing on a particular exercise, find an alternate. It's that simple.

I've grouped the workouts into five categories. They are:

- Beginner Workouts
- Mixed Workouts (negative variations included)
- Negative-only Workouts
- Upper Body Workouts
- Lower Body Workouts

(There's no law that says you can't spend a few weeks just training your upper or lower body!) Many of you will be able to custom tailor your workouts from the master lists in each chapter or the one below. Remember, though, that quality is more important than quantity. Don't perform four biceps exercises in a row and expect to grow big arms. My advice is to work no muscle group with more than three exercises (compound machines counting as two). Two exercises will be sufficient for 95% of you.

Let's start with a complete listing of machines and exercises (see chart on page 91), then review training guidelines briefly before hitting the workouts.

REVIEW OF TRAINING GUIDELINES

1. A workout should consist of no more than fourteen exercises.
2. Choose a weight that will allow about 12

repetitions for the upper body exercises and 15 for the lower.

3. Regardless of how many reps *more* than 12 or 15 you can do on any one day, terminate the exercise *ONLY* at the point of momentary muscular failure. It should technically occur at 12 or 15, but it won't always happen that way.

4. Concentrate on range of motion by letting the machines slowly draw you into the stretched starting positions.

5. Accentuate the lowering or negative/eccentric phase of every repetition by moving at one-half the speed you used to lift the weight.

6. Always move at a slow and controlled speed. Never explode into the weights or move them so quickly that they gain their own momentum.

7. Strength gains are maximized by resting between machines. Cardiovascular and anaerobic endurance gains are maximized by moving rapidly between machines.

8. Once you have reached the 12- or 15-repetition goal on an exercise, increase the weight by about 5% for the next workout. Use

1-, 2½-, and 5-pound weights pinned to the weight stack (insert pin through weight then into weight stack) to make these small changes.

9. Train on Nautilus no more than three times a week. Allow at least 48 hours between workouts.

10. Keep accurate records of everything you do: date, exercise, reps, weight, variations, etc. Seat height should be marked prominently on your card for each machine.

11. Vary your workouts at least every six weeks. This will effectively prevent plateauing and staleness.

12. Always breathe normally. Most will feel comfortable exhaling on the contraction and inhaling on the relaxation (the negative).

WORKOUTS

Beginner

Beginner Workout 1

1. Hip and Back
2. Leg Extension
3. Leg Press
4. Pullover
5. Torso Arm
6. Arm Cross (Double Chest)
7. Incline Press (Double Chest)
8. Lateral Raise (Double Shoulder or free-standing)
9. Overhead Press (Double Shoulder)
10. Biceps Curl (Multi-, Plateloader, or Multi-Exercise)
11. Multi-Exercise Wrist Curls
12. Multi-Exercise Reverse Wrist Curls
13. Abdominal

Beginner Workout 2

1. Hip and Back
2. Leg Extension
3. Leg Curl
4. Behind Neck
5. Torso Arm
6. Rowing Torso
7. Multi-Exercise Triceps Dips
8. Biceps Curls (Multi-, Plateloader, or Multi-Exercise)
9. Multi-Exercise Wrist Curls
10. Multi-Exercise Reverse Wrist Curls
11. Multi-Exercise Calf Raises
12. Abdominal
13. Low Back

Beginner Workout 3

1. Leg Extension
2. Duo Squat
3. Hip Adductor
4. Hip Abductor
5. Pullover
6. Multi-Exercise Chin-Ups
7. Arm Cross
8. Incline Press
9. Biceps Curl (three machines)
10. Multi-Exercise Wrist Curls
11. Four-Way Neck (all four sides)
12. Abdominal

Beginner Workout 4

1. Leg Extension
2. Duo Squat
3. Leg Curl
4. Behind Neck
5. Multi-Exercise Chin-Ups
6. Lateral Raise
7. Overhead Press
8. Rowing Torso
9. Biceps
10. Multi-Exercise Wrist Curls
11. Four-Way Neck
12. Multi-Exercise Calf Raises
13. Abdominal

Beginner Workout 5

1. Hip and Back
2. Leg Extension
3. Leg Curl
4. Multi-Exercise Calf Raise
5. Foot Flexor on Leg Curl
6. Pullover
7. Behind Neck
8. 70° Shoulder
9. 40° Chest/Shoulder

10. 10° Chest
11. Biceps Curl
12. Triceps Extensions (Multi- or Plate-loader)
13. Abdominal

Beginner Workout 6

1. Duo Squat
2. Leg Curl
3. Multi-Exercise Calf Raise
4. Foot Flexor on Leg Curl
5. Pullover
6. Torso Arm
7. 70° Shoulder
8. Incline Press
9. Biceps Curls
10. Abdominal
11. Hip Flexor
12. Low Back

Beginner Workout 7

1. Hip and Back
2. Duo Squat
3. Leg Curl
4. Hip Flexor
5. Adductor
6. Abductor
7. Multi-Exercise Chin-Ups
8. 70° Shoulder
9. Overhead Press (Double Shoulder)
10. Multi-Exercise Triceps Dips
11. Biceps Curl
12. Abdominal
13. Low Back

Beginner Workout 8

1. Hip and Back
2. Leg Extension
3. Leg Curl
4. Adductor
5. Abductor
6. Pullover
7. Torso Arm
8. 70° Shoulder
9. 40° Chest/Shoulder
10. Biceps Curl
11. Abdominal
12. Low Back

Mixed

Mixed Workout 1

1. Hip and Back
2. Leg Extension
3. Leg Press on Compound Leg
4. Adductor
5. Abductor
6. Pullover
7. Negative Multi-Exercise Chin-Ups
8. Arm Cross
9. Negative-only Incline Press
10. Multi-Exercise Triceps Dips
11. Negative-only Multi-Exercise Calf Raise (lift into raised position with help of arms; lower to a count of ten with calves)
12. Abdominal
13. Low Back

Mixed Workout 2

1. Pullover
2. Negative Multi-Exercise Chin-Ups
3. Lateral Raise
4. Rowing Torso
5. Negative-only Multi-Exercise Triceps Dips
6. Leg Extension—Negative-accentuated (lift with two legs, lower with one)
7. Leg Curl—Negative-emphasized (spotter applies extra resistance on the negative phase)
8. Multi-Exercise Calf Raise
9. Foot Flexor on Leg Curl
10. Abdominal
11. Hip Flexor
12. Low Back

Mixed Workout 3

1. Duo Squat Akinetic (set your weight at 50%–75% of what you normally use; swing infimetric bar into place)
2. Leg Extension
3. Leg Curl
4. Adductor
5. Abductor
6. Pullover—Negative-only (use foot pedal or spotter to bring stack into contracted position)

7. Multi-Exercise   Chin-Ups—Negative-only
8. 70° Shoulder
9. 40° Chest/Shoulder
10. Multi-Biceps Machine Curl—Negative-only (bring one lever into contracted position with two arms, lower with one)
11. Multi-Exercise Wrist Curls
12. Abdominal

Mixed Workout 4

1. Duo Squat
2. Leg Extension—Negative-accentuated (raise with both legs, lower with one)
3. Leg Curl
4. Hip Flexor
5. Pullover
6. Negative-only Multi-Exercise Chin-Ups
7. Lateral Raise
8. Overhead Press
9. Negative-only Multi-Exercise Triceps Dips
10. Biceps Curls
11. Multi-Exercise Wrist Curls
12. Abdominal
13. Low Back

Mixed Workout 5

1. Hip and Back
2. Duo Squat
3. Leg Extension—Negative-accentuated
4. Leg Curl—Negative-emphasized
5. Behind Neck
6. Torso Arm—Negative-only (spotter brings bar down into contracted position)
7. 70° Shoulder
8. 10° Chest
9. Multi-Exercise Triceps Dips
10. Multi-Biceps Machine Curls—Negative-only
11. Abdominal
12. Rotary Torso
13. Low Back

Mixed Workout 6

1. Hip and Back
2. Duo Squat
3. Leg Extension—Negative-emphasized

(spotter applies resistance to foot rollers on negative phase)
4. Leg Curl—Negative-accentuated
5. Pullover
6. Multi-Exercise   Chin-Ups—Negative-only
7. Lateral Raise
8. Overhead Press
9. Arm Cross
10. Incline Press—Negative-only
11. Multi-Triceps Machine—Infimetric
12. Multi-Biceps Machine—Infimetric
13. Abdominal

Mixed Workout 7

1. Duo Squat—Infimetric
2. Leg Extension
3. Leg Curl
4. Adductor
5. Abductor
6. Behind Neck
7. Torso Arm—Negative-only (use spotter)
8. 70° Shoulder
9. Arm Cross
10. Multi-Triceps Machine—Infimetric (50% of normal weight load)
11. Abdominal
12. Rotary Torso
13. Low Back

Negative

Negative Workout 1

1. Leg Extension—Negative-accentuated
2. Leg Press (Compound Leg)—Negative-emphasized
3. Leg Curl—Negative-accentuated
4. Multi-Exercise Calf Raise—Negative-only
5. Pullover—Negative-only
6. Multi-Exercise   Chin-Ups—Negative-only
7. Lateral Raise—Negative-only (use a spotter on each arm
8. Overhead Press—Negative-only (use spotter behind machine)
9. Multi-Exercise Triceps Dips—Negative-only

10. Multi-Biceps Machine—Negative-accentuated
11. Abdominal—Negative-only (use spotter)

Negative Workout 2

1. Hip and Back (normal)
2. Leg Extension—Negative-emphasized
3. Leg Press (Compound Leg)—Negative-emphasized
4. Leg Curl—Negative-only (use spotter)
5. Pullover—Negative-emphasized
6. Torso Arm—Negative-only (use spotter)
7. Overhead Press—Negative-only (use spotter)
8. Multi-Exercise Triceps Dips—Negative-emphasized (with hip belt)
9. Multi-Biceps Machine—Negative-only (one arm at a time)
10. Multi-Exercise Calf Raises—Negative-only
11. Abdominal—Negative-only

Negative Workout 3

1. Pullover (normal)
2. Multi-Exercise Chin-Ups—Negative-emphasized (with hip belt)
3. Arm Cross—Negative-emphasized (spotter in front or one at each side)
4. Incline Press—Negative-emphasized (apply extra resistance against foot pedal)
5. 70° Shoulder (normal)
6. Multi-Biceps Machine—Negative-only
7. Leg Extension—Negative-accentuated
8. Leg Curl—Negative-emphasized
9. Multi-Exercise Calf Raises—Negative-only
10. Abdominal (normal)
11. Low Back (normal)

Negative Workout 4

1. Duo Squat (normal)
2. Leg Extension—Negative-emphasized
3. Leg Curl—Negative-accentuated
4. Multi-Exercise Calf Raise—Negative-only
5. Pullover—Negative-only

6. Multi-Exercise Chin-Ups—Negative-emphasized (with hip belt)
7. Overhead Press—Negative-only (with spotter)
8. Arm Cross (normal)
9. Incline Press—Negative-only
10. Multi-Exercise Triceps Dips—Negative-emphasized (with hip belt)
11. Multi-Exercise Machine—Upright Rowing (normal)
12. Abdominal
13. Low Back

Negative Workout 5

1. Hip and Back (normal)
2. Leg Extension—Negative-emphasized
3. Leg Curl—Negative-emphasized
4. Multi-Exercise Calf Raises—Negative-only
5. Behind Neck (normal)
6. Multi-Exercise Chin-Ups—Negative-emphasized (with hip belt)
7. Arm Cross—Negative-emphasized (two spotters if possible)
8. Overhead Press—Negative-only
9. Multi-Exercise Triceps Dips—Negative-emphasized (with hip belt)
10. Multi-Biceps Machine—Negative-only (one arm at a time)
11. Abdominal
12. Rotary Torso

Upper Body

Upper Body Workout 1

1. Pullover
2. Torso Arm
3. Lateral Raise
4. Overhead Press
5. Arm Cross
6. Incline Press
7. Multi-Exercise Triceps Dips
8. Biceps Curl
9. Multi-Exercise Upright Rowing
10. Multi-Exercise Wrist Curl
11. Multi-Exercise Reverse Wrist Curl
12. Abdominal

Upper Body Workout 2

1. Behind Neck
2. Torso Arm
3. 70° Shoulder
4. Rowing Torso
5. 10° Chest
6. Multi-Triceps Infimetric
7. Multi-Biceps Infimetric
8. Multi-Exercise Upright Rowing
9. Multi-Exercise Wrist Curls
10. Multi-Exercise Reverse Wrist Curls

Upper Body Workout 3

1. Pullover
2. Multi-Exercise Chin-Ups
3. Lateral Raise
4. 70° Shoulder
5. Arm Cross
6. Incline Press
7. Triceps Extensions
8. Multi-Exercise Triceps Dips—Negative-only
9. Biceps Curl
10. Upright Rowing (Multi-Exercise)
11. Multi-Exercise Wrist Curls
12. Multi-Exercise Reverse Wrist Curls

Upper Body Workout 4

1. Pullover
2. Behind Neck
3. Multi-Exercise   Chin-Ups—Negative-only
4. Lateral Raise
5. 70° Chest
6. Overhead Press
7. Arm Cross
8. Incline Press
9. Rowing Torso
10. Triceps Extensions
11. Biceps Curls
12. Abdominal

Upper Body Workout 5

1. Behind Neck
2. Pullover
3. Arm Cross
4. Rowing Torso

5. Overhead Press
6. Multi-Exercise Triceps Dips
7. Multi-Exercise Upright Rowing
8. Biceps Curls
9. Multi-Exercise Wrist Curls
10. Multi-Exercise Reverse Wrist Curls
11. Abdominal
12. Low Back

Lower Body

Lower Body Workout 1

1. Duo Squat
2. Leg Extension
3. Leg Curl
4. Hip Flexor
5. Adductor
6. Abductor
7. Multi-Exercise Calf Raise
8. Foot Flexor on Leg Curl
9. Abdominal
10. Rotary Torso
11. Low Back

Lower Body Workout 2

1. Hip and Back
2. Leg Extension
3. Duo Squat
4. Leg Curl
5. Adductor
6. Abductor
7. Multi-Exercise Calf Raise
8. Foot Flexor on Leg Curl
9. Abdominal
10. Hip Flexor
11. Low Back

Lower Body Workout 3

1. Hip and Back
2. Duo Squat
3. Leg Curl
4. Leg Extension
5. Hip Flexor
6. Multi-Exercise Calf Raise
7. Foot Flexor on Leg Curl
8. Adductor
9. Abductor

10. Abdominal
11. Rotary Torso
12. Low Back

FINAL TRAINING NOTE

Advanced Nautilus users may find the following training method quite productive:

1. Get two weight stack pins ready and a capable trainer to use them.

2. Place the first pin about three plates heavier than your usual training weight.

3. Place the second pin in the plate above the first.

4. Attempt three repetitions with perfect form at the unusually high starting weight. If you can't do this, start only two plates above normal.

5. Have the spotter immediately pull the pin out of the bottom plate after the three reps and jump it over the second pin to the plate above that.

6. Attempt another three perfect reps with the weight that the second pin had set.

7. After these three reps, the trainer again jumps the pin upward and you start working with the weight that he/she set with the first pin.

8. Keep training as your spotter jumps the pins upward and over each other to the very first plate—if you can last that long! Don't use this technique more than twice a workout—it's brutally hard.

11
AEROBIC TRAINING STRATEGIES

If you're a graduate of the Mark Twain School of Exercise—whenever he felt the urge to exercise he lay down and waited for it to pass—this chapter's not for you.

Aerobic exercise does several things that Nautilus can't, primary among them being its contribution to weight control. As you remember from Chapter 2, Nautilus involves highly anaerobic exercise, and the anaerobic system cannot use fat as an energy source. The only way to cause your body to break down fat is to crank up the aerobic system and keep it going for at least 30 minutes. The ideal reshaping program, for both men and women, includes Nautilus for muscle toning or building and aerobics for fat reduction.

THE NEED FOR AEROBICS

Aerobics also appear to have a much stronger effect than anaerobics (Nautilus) on overall cardiovascular health. Though there is still much research to do, aerobic exercise seems to improve heart function and blood lipids (fats) more effectively than Nautilus.

High density lipids (HDL), the "good" form of cholesterol that rids the blood vessels of "bad" cholesterol deposits, is found in its highest levels in aerobic athletes.

From research on both humans and animals at several major universities, it appears that aerobic training slows the aging process. Based upon the work of some graduate student named Wolf, researchers at The University of Texas showed that lifelong treadmill training keeps rats at peak motor efficiency. Old rats, trained aerobically throughout their lives, were found to possess the reaction times and motor abilities of healthy, young rats! The same finding held true in another Texas study of 70–80 year old handball/paddleball players—their reaction times matched those of healthy college students!

Finally, aerobic fitness forms the base for stamina and endurance in most of life's activities. After all, how many things do you start that are over and done with in 60 seconds, and are therefore purely anaerobic?

Safe and effective aerobic exercise is based on the answers to four questions:

- What types of exercise are aerobic?
- What intensity of exercise is required?
- How long must each workout last?
- How often must I train aerobically?

These are the four components of an exercise prescription: type, intensity, duration, and frequency. Let's address these first then move on to training strategies and workout for our aerobic choices.

TYPES OF EXERCISE

To qualify as aerobic, an exercise must make rhythmic and repetitive use of the major muscle groups for at least 10 minutes. High heart rate is not enough, for many nonaerobic activities can raise your heart rate. Here are your best choices.

Jogging/Running

Among the best choices for aerobic benefits, but a risky and dangerous activity. Running offers the perfect example of what aerobics should and shouldn't be. The good part is the rhythmic and repetitive use of the large muscle groups in the front and back thighs and the buttocks. Long jogs/runs are more than 90% fueled by the aerobic system. The bad news: the major orthopedic stress that running causes in your feet/ankles/shins/knees/thighs/hips/lower back. Landing with the force of two-to-three times your body weight, more than a thousand times each mile, does wonders for your medical bills.

Witness: a well-known New Jersey orthopedic surgeon recently disagreed with me in print over my advice in a previous article to leave running to faucets. After telling the reporter who interviewed him that I had greatly exaggerated runners' injury problems, he told the same gentleman that more than 60% of his patients were runners!

The incidence of running injuries can be reduced but never totally eliminated. Your weapons are proper stretching and strength training, the right choices of footwear and running surfaces, and a limit on mileage. Stretching and strength training are covered

right here. Footwear should be selected at a store that specializes in running shoes and is staffed by knowledgeable runners. Concrete is to be avoided at all costs, and the upper limit on miles, if you're not training for a marathon, should be about four to five a day.

Swimming

Along with cross-country (X-C) skiing, it's the best in aerobics. Rhythmic and repetitive use of the major muscles *is* possible without impact forces of several hundred pounds!

Swimming offers the added benefit of a watery medium to reduce heat stress. Since water is an excellent "thermal conductor," you won't have to deal with the problems of heat shock or stroke. Make sure to drink fluids before and after swimming, though—you'll sweat while swimming but won't notice it.

The only recurring injuries from swimming are "breast stroker knee" and "swimmer's shoulder." The latter is a tendinitis problem which is found mostly in freestylers who swim 5,000 meters a day and up. The former results from the "whip kick," a propulsive leg action in the breast stroke which asks the knee, a hinge joint, to rotate. Both problems are rare in recreational fitness swimmers.

Cross-Country Skiing

Combine the sliding motions of the legs and the poling action of the arms and you've got a tremendous aerobic conditioner without any impact forces. Since few of your muscles get to rest during X-C skiing, you'll see the absolute quickest training gains from this activity. The highest aerobic capacities (Max VO_2) found in the world are from Scandinavian X-C skiers.

No, I'm not crazy. I don't expect all of you to head off to Norway for aerobic exercise. For the majority of you that don't live in the cold North, a device known as the Nordic Ski Track brings you indoor X-C skiing. Found in an increasing number of fitness centers and homes (costing less than $600), the Nordic Track lets you stride and pole just as you would on snow. If you're hunting for a center to join, or creating a home gym, ask about the Nordic. The cost factor? Add up what all those visits to the orthopedic surgeon and running shoe store cost!

Cycling

Cycling is a fine aerobic activity, though not as effective as swimming or X-C skiing. Many people are dragging out the old exercise bike to pedal away the six o'clock news, a wonderful way to fit aerobics into your lifestyle. Indoor cycling offers the major advantages of safety and the ability to set a specific workload and pedaling rate. Aerobics shouldn't be any different than Nautilus—could you ever improve your stength without feedback as to reps and plates? Indoor bikes can give you accurate feedback, enabling you to progress your aerobic training just as well as your strength training.

The major problems with outdoor cycling are, of course, safety and the inability (in most places) to put together a solid 20 minutes of pedaling. With hills and traffic conditions, many outdoor rides turn out to include too much coasting and stopping. If you live in an area which allows uninterrupted riding, and you've got a good, safe bike, get to it!

Rowing

Like X-C skiing and swimming, rowing is a whole-body activity. Since the arms and back must work along with the lower body, the aerobic benefits will be broader and possibly greater than with lower-body-only aerobic activities. Expect to pay at least $150 for an acceptable home rowing machine, though the best models will run about $300.

Aerobic Dancing

If the choreographer knows his/her stuff (meaning exercise physiology as well as dancing), aerobic dancing can be a fun and effective training choice. Unfortunately, a huge percentage of these programs are just not aerobic.

Remember why Nautilus is mostly anaerobic exercise? It's the switching back and forth between muscles that does it. A muscle must be contracting rhythmically and repetitively for at least five or six minutes before its aerobic system is fully turned on. Nautilus, and most aerobic dance programs, switch rapidly between muscles and elevate heart rate without ever making the exercise aerobic.

What to look for in an aerobic dancing program? The exercises/dance steps must keep the same, large muscles of the lower body working continuously for 15 minutes or more. There's no way around it: you're going to do a great deal of jogging and kicking. The session should start with a 10–15 minute warm-up, have a 20–30 minute intense, aerobic phase, then close with a 10–15 minute cool-down. The instructor must continually watch and correct poor form. The classes not to sign up for are those where the instructor is too busy admiring herself in the mirror to attend to her class's safety. I've witnessed several spectacles where the instructor danced merrily away while her class twisted and threw their bodies into oblivion. Insist on viewing a complete class before signing or paying.

Jump Rope

Chances are you'll have to build up gradually to get in your 20 minutes of exercise, but jump rope is a fine aerobic choice. Don't believe everything you've heard about it, for one minute of jumping is *not* the equivalent of five miles of running (or some such nonsense). It *is* effective and aerobic, however.

As I'll show you in more detail in a moment, you can build jumping time through a combination of jumping and resting. As you progress, you'll jump more and rest less. It won't take long to get you to the 15–20 minute level.

Minitrampolines/Rebounders

These offer most of the benefits of running without any of the medical/orthopedic risks. I really like these inexpensive devices, for with a little bit of practice, you can get aerobic intensity, indoors, at low cost. Many beginners have trouble getting their heart rates into their "training zones" (see below), but they quickly learn that faster stepping and higher knee lift is all they need. I think you'll be pleasantly surprised if you've never tried one of these.

INTENSITY AND DURATION OF EXERCISE

Good news—you won't have to work to momentary muscular failure for maximal aerobic training gains. In fact, the recommended range of intensity for aerobics is 70%-85% of your maximal heart rate. Working out at a higher intensity will bring you only minimally faster results and presents greater health dangers. There's literally no need to sweat up a storm and go to failure with aerobics.

Finding your personal training zone requires the use of a simple equation known as the *Karvonen Formula*. By taking into consideration your age, resting heart rate, and desired target intensity, the formula gives you an accurate pulse rate to shoot for. Obtain your resting heart rate about five minutes after awakening in the morning. You may use the carotid artery along the windpipe in your neck or the radial artery along the thumb side of your wrist. Count for 60 seconds if you like, but a 15-second count multiplied by four is just as accurate. If you're in fairly good shape, use 70% or 0.7 as your target intensity. (That's 70% of your maximum heart rate.) Just starting out? Try 60% or 0.6. Superfit? Use 0.8 or

80%. The equation and an example to follow are at the bottom of the page.

Your target zone will be ten beats on either side of the target number, in this case 145–165 beats per minute.

After a five-to-ten-minute warm-up, your pulse should be gradually elevated into your target zone. The goal is 20 minutes of target zone aerobics, but remember that fat metabolism doesn't really get rolling until you've hit the 30-minute mark. Keep a close watch on your pulse by stopping for 10 or 15 second intervals during the 20-minute phase. Use the carotid or radial arteries (don't press too hard) and multiply by six or four to get your heart rate. Pulse too low? Pick it up. Pulse too high? Ease off—the benefits aren't much greater but the dangers are.

Follow your aerobic phase with a cool-down that gradually brings your pulse back toward resting level. Five or ten minutes of light exercise is usually sufficient. See Chapter 12 for more specific warm-up and cool-down ideas.

FREQUENCY OF TRAINING

How often you train aerobically depends on how hard you train. Ideally, your weekly training schedule would include five days of aerobics and two or three Nautilus workouts. The aerobics would include a warm-up and cool-down and about 30 minutes of training zone exercise. The Nautilus workouts should last between 20 and 30 minutes, and should be separated from the aerobics by several hours. If your aerobic training goes much

Target Heart Rate = (220 minus **Your Age** minus **Resting Heart Rate**) times 0.7 plus **Resting Heart Rate**

Age: 30   **Resting Heart Rate:** 75   **Target Intensity:** 0.7 (70%)

Target Heart Rate = (220 − 30 − 75) × 0.7 + 75
= (115   ) × 0.7 + 75
= 80.5 + 75 = 155.5

beyond 30 minutes at 70% intensity, you should consider cutting back to four a week.

Overtraining is the most frequent cause of poor results from exercise. If you're running ten miles a day, six days a week, don't expect to get a great deal out of Nautilus. That kind of distance keeps your body in a constantly broken-down state, and prevents large-scale muscle growth. I've had great success, though, with recreational runners who cut back to five, faster miles a day (higher quality, lower quantity), four days a week. They found both aerobic and Nautilus benefits to be greater than before.

The minimum amount of exercise that will train you is two aerobic and two Nautilus workouts a week. It is best to perform them on alternate days so that neither interferes with the other. If they must be done on the same day, keep them several hours apart. If they must be done in one workout, do Nautilus first if strength and muscle are your primary goal, aerobics first if otherwise. *Never strength train immediately before skill training,* for a tired body will perform very differently than a rested one. Skill practice such as baseball batting, basketball shooting, or golf should always precede strength training.

TRAINING TIPS AND WORKOUTS

There's a lot more to aerobic training than 20 boring minutes of continuous exercise. Your aerobic workouts can and should make use of the three major training techniques:

- Long, slow distance (LSD) or Overdistance
- Fartlek or Speedplay
- Interval Training

Overdistance—LSD

Just as the name suggests, overdistance is a technique that involves low-intensity work over longer-than-usual distances. Athletes in aerobic sports always begin a new season with overdistance training. It establishes a good, solid aerobic base upon which quality, anaerobic power, and sprinting can later be developed.

Overdistance applies best to running, swimming, and cycling. Keep the intensity low and maximize distance. Some of the other aerobic choices, like rope jumping and rowing, are better suited to interval training (see below).

Speedplay/Fartlek

This technique originated in Scandinavia many years back, and involves alternation between hard and easy work during one continuous exercise bout. As an example, a swimmer might cover a 1,000-yard distance by alternating two easy laps with two hard laps. A runner might similarly sprint the straights on a track and jog the curves. A rope jumper might alternate 30 seconds of a 140-turns-per-minute pace with 30 seconds of a 100-turns pace. Well, you get the idea . . . .

Speedplay brings fun to otherwise boring overdistance work, and can be infinitely varied. Check out this example for an interest-maintaining 1,000-yard (40-lap) swim:

Easy Laps	Hard Laps	Total Yards
1	1	50
2	2	150
3	3	300
4	4	500
4	4	700
3	3	850
2	2	950
1	1	1,000

Interval Training

The simple process of alternating exercise bouts with rest periods, called *interval training,* is the single most important training innovation in the last 30 years. Anyone, from beginner to world record-holder, in any exercise or sport, can use interval training.

It's the manipulation of the exercise and rest periods that makes interval training so valuable. If you're just beginning a program, you will keep the rest intervals long and the exercise bouts brief. As your fitness level improves, the work/rest ratio changes—more exercise, less rest. Before you realize it you'll be ready for overdistance and speedplay training. If you're an athlete, you'll use interval training (intervals) to develop speed, power, and endurance.

Writing Your Interval Training Program

Let's look at the guidelines for writing a personalized interval training prescription, an ITP. Your prescription has four components:

- the number of repetitions
- the distance or exercise time
- the amount of rest between reps
- the type of rest between reps

A swimmer's ITP might look something like this:

[10 × 100 freestyle, 60 seconds active rest]

- swim 100 yards a total of ten times
- rest for 60 seconds between each 100
- do some light stretching or swimming during the 60-second rest interval

Number of Repetitions

The usual range is 4–20. Most frequently, an ITP will specify 8–12 reps. Lower numbers of reps are usually called for if the quality of the exercise is high, such as season-ending sprint training. Higher reps are usually employed earlier in the season with lower intensity exercise.

Distance or Exercise Time

This variable may be set as either a distance to run/swim/etc., or a time to exercise, i.e., run two minutes and rest 30 seconds or run 10 × 800. The distance/time you choose depends entirely on what you're training for. A beginner may only be capable of 15 seconds of rope jumping. That's fine, for as you can see in the table on page 105, you can write an ITP that alternates 15 seconds of jumping with 45 seconds or more of rest. Repeat eight times and you've jumped for two minutes! Other examples: a 100-yard freestyle swimmer will usually choose intervals in the 50- to 200-yard or 30-second-to-two-minute range. An 800-meter runner might work within the 200–1,500-meter and 30-second-to-four-minute range. "Doing" intervals at distances longer than those you compete at helps build the stamina to finish your event strongly.

There's no limit to distance or exercise time in an ITP. I'll absolutely never forget the Saturday morning workout when my coach sat back with a half-finished book and ordered 4 × 1,650 swims on 20 minutes! ("On 20 minutes" means that a new swim is started every 20 minutes. If one swim takes 18:15, it is followed by 1:45 of rest before the next is begun.)

Amount of Rest between Reps

This variable is determined either by the quality of work you want to do or your fitness level. Beginners will invariably want to use long rest intervals so that they can maximize the amount of exercise that can be tolerated. The work/rest ratio can be 1/4 or higher—60 seconds of rest to 15 seconds of exercise. Athletes will maximize rest intervals when the speed or quality of the exercise bout must be high. At the end of a season, for example, runners might try to run each of six 200-meter sprints at 90% of maximum. This will require at least two minutes of rest between reps. During the early season, when distance and an aerobic base are more important, they might run 10 × 200 with only 30 seconds of rest.

Here's a brief summary for athletes:

- Early season: High work/rest ratio. Run 800, walk 100.
- Midseason: Medium work/rest ratio. Run 400, walk 400.
- Late season: Low work/rest ratio. Run 200, walk 800.

Types of Rest between Reps

All rest is not created equal. Depending again on what athletic events you may be training for, rest will be either *active* or *inactive*.

Athletes in speed and power events depend heavily upon their stored *phosphagens* (ATP and CP). If they remain totally inactive during their rest intervals, the ATP–CP system can recharge fully and allow full-speed-ahead on the next repetition. A series of reps with inactive rest will nicely train your ATP–CP system and let you run/swim/etc. each rep with high quality. Beginners will want to use inactive rest because the extra boost of stored ATP and CP will keep them going a bit longer.

Should you perform light exercise during each rest interval (active rest) you'll prevent the ATP–CP system from fully recharging. This is *exactly* what the anaerobic event athlete wants, however. The shortage of stored ATP and CP places extra stress on the anaerobic system, and is excellent for athletes whose events last between 20 seconds and three-to-four minutes.

Interval training can adapt to just about any aerobic choice you make. By interspersing periodic rest intervals, lactate levels can be kept from skyrocketing and more high-quality work can be performed. Your imagination is the only limit to interval training!

SWIMMING: A SEASON'S STRATEGY

Early Season Training

Primarily LSD (long, slow distance). Fill your swim time with a few long, easy swims, broken up by some kicking drills. Break the boredom of overdistance training by varying breathing patterns and including some Fartlek (speedplay) work. Utilize but don't overdo pulling drills (legs are buoyed and arms do all the work). Use all four strokes (freestyle, back, breast, and butterfly), but make sure at least 50% of your distance is free.

EARLY SEASON 60-MINUTE WORKOUT

Warmup—400 swim, 50 free, 50 breast
    Swim—1,000 free, first 500 breathe every 4 strokes, second 500 every 3
      Kick—400 IM (100 each of fly, back, whip, flutter)
    Swim—600 free, two laps easy, one lap hard

Midseason Training

Primarily interval training with short rest. Get in at least two main sets a workout, with at least eight repeats of longer-than-race-distance swims, and not more than 45 seconds of rest. If you compete at 200 yards, a sample set would be eight 300s. Concentrate on distance per stroke rather than speed. Stretch out and still enjoy the swims. Make some sets all one stroke, some individual medley.

MIDSEASON 60-MINUTE WORKOUT

Warm-up—500 swim (100 fly, 100 back, 100 breast, 200 free)
    Swim—8 × 200 free, 30 seconds rest, breathing every third stroke. *Descending Set:* get progressively faster from #1 to #8. (Inactive rest)
    Kick—8 × 100 flutter, 45 seconds rest
    Swim—8 × 200 Individual Medley, 45 seconds rest
    Swim—Easy 200 cooldown

Late Season Training

You're still using interval training, but you'll swim fewer reps, with more rest, at faster speeds. This is the up-the-quality, lower-the-quantity phase of training. Keep thinking about technique, but speed is of the essence. Try "broken swims" to accustom your body to fast swimming (swim a 200, but rest 10 seconds between each 50; this allows extra-fast swimming).

LATE-SEASON 60-MINUTE WORKOUT

Warm-up—300 swim, 100 kick, 200 swim (all freestyle)
    Swim—5 × 200, 60-second rest (inactive), descending from #1–#5, stroke of your choice
    Kick—4 × 100, 60 seconds rest, flutter
    Swim—6 × 200 IM, 60 seconds rest, *broken* with 10-second rest at each 50 (inactive)
    Swim—500 easy, mixed strokes

Precompetition Swimming

Make sure your quantity of swimming and strength training is considerably reduced over the last three weeks before competition. Each workout should contain no more than 600 yards of hard swimming in the last week or two. Get plenty of sleep and eat well. Good luck!

JUMPING ROPE THE INTERVAL WAY

Try this four-month plan for jumping rope through interval training.

Guidelines

1. Setting correct rope length: Stand on the middle of the rope—the handles should just reach your armpits. Tie knots near the handles to shorten the rope.
2. Keep jumping height low, the knees flexible and slightly bent, and the wrists close to the body.
3. Jump at a rate of about 100 per minute.
4. Watch your pulse! Keep it *in* the training zone, not *above*.

Week	Jump Time (seconds)	Rest Time (seconds)	Reps	Total Daily (minutes)
1	15	45	8	2
2	15	30	12	3.0
3	15	15	12	3.0
4	30	30	8	4.0
5	30	15	8	4.0
6	45	20	8	6.0
7	60	30	7	7.0
8	90	30	6	9.0
9	120	60	5	10.0
10	150	60	5	12.5
11	180	60	5	15.0
12	240	60	4	16.0
13	360	60	3	18.0
14	420	60	3	21.0
15	480	60	3	24.0

12

WARM-UPS, STRETCHES, COOL-DOWNS—NOT TO BE AVOIDED!

Warm-ups, stretching exercises, and cool-downs are taken too lightly by most people, and that's a shame. They play a key role both in improving training results and reducing injury risks. You've been told for years by Nautilus that a pre-workout warm-up isn't necessary. The first few reps on each machine are "supposed" to be sufficient warm-up. It just ain't so.

Jumping into a high-intensity Nautilus workout offers great risk to the heart. Medically, such a practice is called sudden, strenuous exercise—SSE—and it's been shown to cause several serious types of heart dysfunction. Don't even risk such danger. Precede every Nautilus workout with warm-up exercise and a stretching program.

And in just that order, too. Light exercise should always *precede* flexibility work to reduce the danger of stretching a cold muscle. Think of muscle as taffy. The only way to stretch taffy is to warm it up. Try stretching or bending cold taffy and it will break. The analogy isn't far from accurate.

THE WARM-UP

The absolute best warm-up exercise is walking. Begin walking at a slow pace with an easy and short arm swing. Step up both the pace and the arm swing gradually over a five-to-ten-minute period. You should finish with a brisk pace and a vigorous arm swing. Don't, however, break into a run. You may ease down for a minute or so at this point.

If walking is impossible (no indoor track or treadmill, uncooperative weather conditions), you've got several alternatives. An accelerating-pace exercise bicycle ride works well. So does an accelerating-pace bounce on a minitrampoline. Easy jumping jacks (on carpet, with good athletic footwear) will turn the trick, too. Whatever you choose, start slowly and build slowly. Give your body time to get ready for high-intensity work.

STRETCHING

Following the warm-up, move into a

stretching routine. Some Nautilus machines *will* improve flexibility, but most will, at best, only maintain you. To improve your flexibility you'll need to stretch.

The program on pages 108–111 was carefully designed to effectively stretch specific muscles while placing as little stress as possible on other parts of the body. Permanent gains in flexibility will only come from static or stationary stretching. You should hold a stretched position for at least 20 seconds, for it takes that long to permanently lengthen the so-called *plastic element*—the one that makes you tight or flexible.

Bouncing or "ballistic" stretching can only lengthen the *elastic element,* which, like a rubber band, snaps right back to its original length. Bouncing can also be extremely destructive to connective tissue and muscle.

Follow the instructions for each stretch, taking yourself into a pain-free position. Hold it for 20 seconds, release, shake out, then repeat at a slightly greater stretch. Do this at least three times.

Perform one stretch from each of the categories. If you can make the time, stretch after the workout as well as before. You should even experiment with only stretching afterwards if your time is limited.

THE COOL-DOWN

Your body will physiologically appreciate light exercise after a workout. By keeping the muscles contracting, blood flow back to the heart is ensured and blood cannot "pool" in the arms or legs. At the same time, the constant flow of blood helps wash lactic acid out of the muscles and may also prevent next-day soreness. Since Nautilus exercise is at least 50% anaerobic, you can expect lots of lactic acid!

Cool-down exercises are much like warm-up choices—walking, cycling, rebounding. Of course, you won't do them at an accelerating pace now. Try a ten minute cool-down walk after your next Nautilus workout—you'll love it.

The Stretching Program

Body Part	Exercise
Neck	Lateral Rotation
Upper Back	Meditation Sit
Shoulders	Rear Deltoid Stretch, Front Deltoid Stretch
Torso	Side Bends
Pectoralis	Iron Cross
Groin	One-Leg Abduction, Two-Leg Abduction
Quadriceps	Standing Quad Stretch, Kneeling Quad Stretch
Hamstrings	Half-Lotus Ham Stretch, Two-Leg Hamstring Stretch
Calves	Wall Stretch

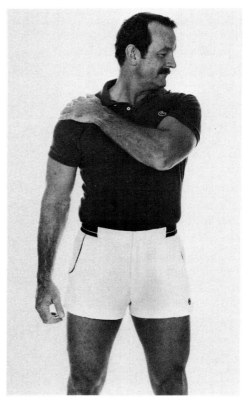

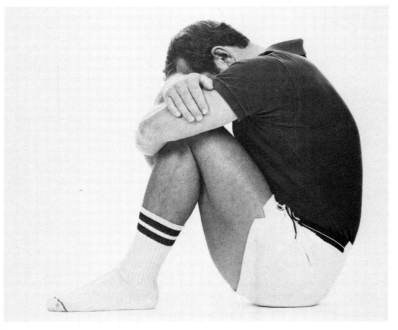

Above, Left:
Lateral Rotation. Place one arm on the opposite shoulder while rotating the head in the opposite direction.

Above, right:
Meditation Sit. Cross your arms over your knees, head down, and stretch the upper back and shoulders.

Below, left:
Rear Deltoid Stretch. Pull one arm across the chest with the other to stretch the back of the shoulder.

Below, right:
Front Deltoid Stretch. Stand facing the wall, and place your arm against the wall, parallel to floor. Turn slowly away from the wall to stretch front deltoid and pectoralis.

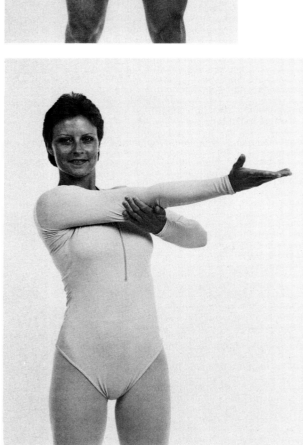

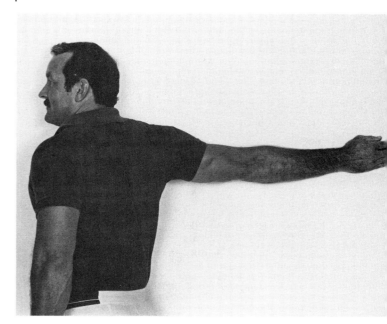

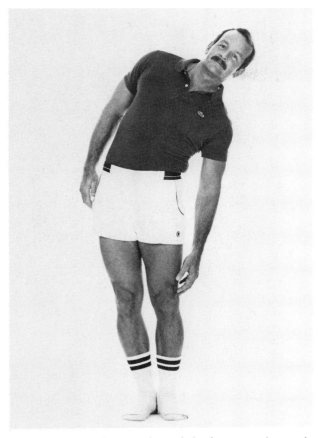

Side Bends. Bend in a right-to-left plane (not forward or backward), keeping the hands close to the sides. Keep the stomach tucked in and the back flat.

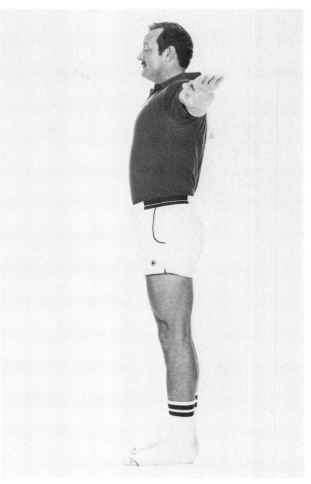

Iron Cross. Raise both arms to the side and draw back as far as possible. Minimize arching of the back.

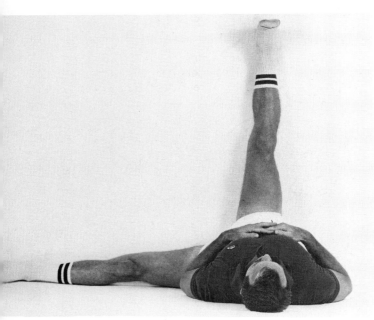

One-Leg Abduction. Lay at the base of the wall with both feet pointing toward the ceiling. Slowly inch one leg downward, reaching the floor if possible.

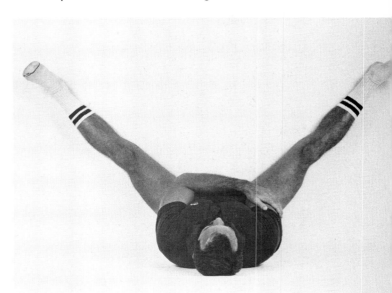

Two-Leg Abduction. Start with both legs together, pointing toward the ceiling. Bring both legs downward simultaneously to stretch the groin.

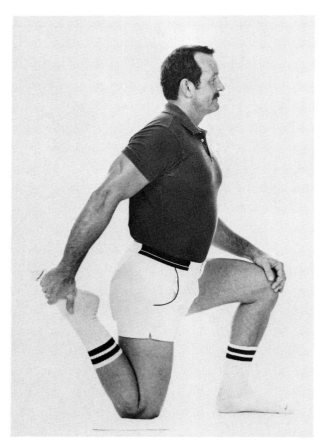

Kneeling Quad Stretch. With a cushion under the knee resting on the floor, grasp the front of the foot and pull it slowly up toward the buttocks. Keep the other foot roughly beneath its knee. Do not arch back.

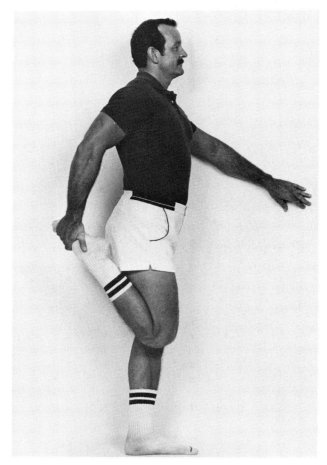

Standing Quad Stretch. Stabilizing against a wall or a chair, grasp the top of one foot and pull it up toward the buttocks. Initially, keep the knees together. If you can easily touch the heel to your buttocks, gradually pull the upper leg directly backward to stretch quads from the hip joint.

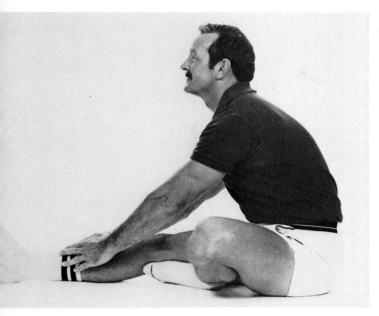

Half-Lotus Ham Stretch. Sit forward with your head up and your back as straight as possible. Keep one leg straight out in front of you, and bend the other leg. Grasp and hold the straight leg at a point where you just begin to feel a stretch in the hamstrings. Always press forward with the chest; never curl your back over toward the feet (this really places stress on the lower back).

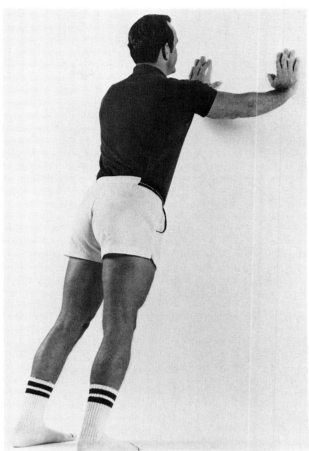

Wall Stretch. Stand about three feet from the wall, point toes slightly inward, and lean forward until hands press against the wall. Keep heels down to stretch the calves. Move your feet slowly backward to increase the stretch.

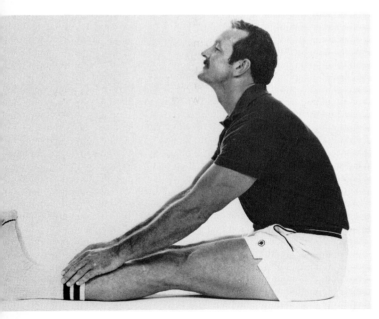

Two-Leg Ham Stretch. Identical to Half-Lotus but both legs are extended. Be careful with your back!

APPENDIX I:
ENERGY EXPENDITURE IN HOUSEHOLD, RECREATIONAL, AND SPORT ACTIVITIES

(in kcal · min⁻¹)

ACTIVITY	kcal·min⁻¹·kg⁻¹	kg 50 lb 110	53 117	56 123	59 130	62 137	65 143	68 150
Archery	0.065	3.3	3.4	3.6	3.8	4.0	4.2	4.4
Badminton	0.097	4.9	5.1	5.4	5.7	6.0	6.3	6.6
Bakery, general (F)	0.035	1.8	1.9	2.0	2.1	2.2	2.3	2.4
Basketball	0.138	6.9	7.3	7.7	8.1	8.6	9.0	9.4
Billiards	0.042	2.1	2.2	2.4	2.5	2.6	2.7	2.9
Bookbinding	0.038	1.9	2.0	2.1	2.2	2.4	2.5	2.6
Boxing								
in ring	0.222	6.9	7.3	7.7	8.1	8.6	9.0	9.4
sparring	0.138	11.1	11.8	12.4	13.1	13.8	14.4	15.1
Canoeing								
leisure	0.044	2.2	2.3	2.5	2.6	2.7	2.9	3.0
racing	0.103	5.2	5.5	5.8	6.1	6.4	6.7	7.0
Card playing	0.025	1.3	1.3	1.4	1.5	1.6	1.6	1.7
Carpentry, general	0.052	2.6	2.8	2.9	3.1	3.2	3.4	3.5
Carpet sweeping (F)	0.045	2.3	2.4	2.5	2.7	2.8	2.9	3.1
Carpet sweeping (M)	0.048	2.4	2.5	2.7	2.8	3.0	3.1	3.3
Circuit-training	0.185	9.3	9.8	10.4	10.9	11.5	12.0	12.6
Cleaning (F)	0.062	3.1	3.3	3.5	3.7	3.8	4.0	4.2
Cleaning (M)	0.058	2.9	3.1	3.2	3.4	3.6	3.8	3.9
Climbing hills								
with no load	0.121	6.1	6.4	6.8	7.1	7.5	7.9	8.2
with 5-kg load	0.129	6.5	6.8	7.2	7.6	8.0	8.4	8.8
with 10-kg load	0.140	7.0	7.4	7.8	8.3	8.7	9.1	9.5
with 20-kg load	0.147	7.4	7.8	8.2	8.7	9.1	9.6	10.0
Coal mining								
drilling coal, rock	0.094	4.7	5.0	5.3	5.5	5.8	6.1	6.4
erecting supports	0.088	4.4	4.7	4.9	5.2	5.5	5.7	6.0
shoveling coal	0.108	5.4	5.7	6.0	6.4	6.7	7.0	7.3
Cooking (F)	0.045	2.3	2.4	2.5	2.7	2.8	2.9	3.1
Cooking (M)	0.048	2.4	2.5	2.7	2.8	3.0	3.1	3.3
Cricket								
batting	0.083	4.2	4.4	4.6	4.9	5.1	5.4	5.6
bowling	0.090	4.5	4.8	5.0	5.3	5.6	5.9	6.1

From *Exercise Physiology: Energy, Nutrition, and Human Performance* by W. McArdle, F. I. Katch, and V. L. Katch. © 1981 Lea and Febiger. Reprinted by permission of Lea and Febiger. *NOTE:* The second column (kcal · min⁻¹ · kg⁻¹) represents the amount of calories expended in one minute. To measure your energy expenditure, first locate your weight for kilograms or pounds at the top, and follow down that column to the specific activity. All figures in that column represent the total number of calories expended in one minute.

71 157	74 163	77 170	80 176	83 183	86 190	89 196	92 203	95 209	98 216
4.6	4.8	5.0	5.2	5.4	5.6	5.8	6.0	6.2	6.4
6.9	7.2	7.5	7.8	8.1	8.3	8.6	8.9	9.2	9.5
2.5	2.6	2.7	2.8	2.9	3.0	3.1	3.2	3.3	3.4
9.8	10.2	10.6	11.0	11.5	11.9	12.3	12.7	13.1	13.5
3.0	3.1	3.2	3.4	3.5	3.6	3.7	3.9	4.0	4.1
2.7	2.8	2.9	3.0	3.2	3.3	3.4	3.5	3.6	3.7
9.8	10.2	10.6	11.0	11.5	11.9	12.3	12.7	13.1	13.5
15.8	16.4	17.1	17.8	18.4	19.1	19.8	20.4	21.1	21.8
3.1	3.3	3.4	3.5	3.7	3.8	3.9	4.0	4.2	4.3
7.3	7.6	7.9	8.2	8.5	8.9	9.2	9.5	9.8	10.1
1.8	1.9	1.9	2.0	2.1	2.2	2.2	2.3	2.4	2.5
3.7	3.8	4.0	4.2	4.3	4.5	4.6	4.8	4.9	5.1
3.2	3.3	3.5	3.6	3.7	3.9	4.0	4.1	4.3	4.4
3.4	3.6	3.7	3.8	4.0	4.1	4.3	4.4	4.6	4.7
13.1	13.7	14.2	14.8	15.4	15.9	16.5	17.0	17.6	18.1
4.4	4.6	4.8	5.0	5.1	5.3	5.5	5.7	5.9	6.1
4.1	4.3	4.5	4.6	4.8	5.0	5.2	5.3	5.5	5.7
8.6	9.0	9.3	9.7	10.0	10.4	10.8	11.1	11.5	11.9
9.2	9.5	9.9	10.3	10.7	11.1	11.5	11.9	12.3	12.6
9.9	10.4	10.8	11.2	11.6	12.0	12.5	12.9	13.3	13.7
10.4	10.9	11.3	11.8	12.2	12.6	13.1	13.5	14.0	14.4
6.7	7.0	7.2	7.5	7.8	8.1	8.4	8.6	8.9	9.2
6.2	6.5	6.8	7.0	7.3	7.6	7.8	8.1	8.4	8.6
7.7	8.0	8.3	8.6	9.0	9.3	9.6	9.9	10.3	10.6
3.2	3.3	3.5	3.6	3.7	3.9	4.0	4.1	4.3	4.4
3.4	3.6	3.7	3.8	4.0	4.1	4.3	4.4	4.6	4.7
5.9	6.1	6.4	6.6	6.9	7.1	7.4	7.6	7.9	8.1
6.4	6.7	6.9	7.2	7.5	7.7	8.0	8.3	8.6	8.8

ACTIVITY	kcal·min⁻¹·kg⁻¹	kg / lb	50 / 110	53 / 117	56 / 123	59 / 130	62 / 137	65 / 143	68 / 150
Croquet	0.059		3.0	3.1	3.3	3.5	3.7	3.8	4.0
Cycling									
leisure, 5.5 mph	0.064		3.2	3.4	3.6	3.8	4.0	4.2	4.4
leisure, 9.4 mph	0.100		5.0	5.3	5.6	5.9	6.2	6.5	6.8
racing	0.169		8.5	9.0	9.5	10.0	10.5	11.0	11.5
Dancing									
ballroom	0.051		2.6	2.7	2.9	3.0	3.2	3.3	3.5
choreographed			8.4	8.9	9.4	9.9	10.4	10.9	11.4
"twist," "wiggle"	0.168		5.2	5.5	5.8	6.1	6.4	6.7	7.0
Digging trenches	0.145		7.3	7.7	8.1	8.6	9.0	9.4	9.9
Drawing (standing)	0.036		1.8	1.9	2.0	2.1	2.2	2.3	2.4
Eating (sitting)	0.023		1.2	1.2	1.3	1.4	1.4	1.5	1.6
Electrical work	0.058		2.9	3.1	3.2	3.4	3.6	3.8	3.9
Farming									
barn cleaning	0.135		6.8	7.2	7.6	8.0	8.4	8.8	9.2
driving harvester	0.040		2.0	2.1	2.2	2.4	2.5	2.6	2.7
driving tractor	0.037		1.9	2.0	2.1	2.2	2.3	2.4	2.5
feeding cattle	0.085		4.3	4.5	4.8	5.0	5.3	5.5	5.8
feeding animals	0.065		3.3	3.4	3.6	3.8	4.0	4.2	4.4
forking straw bales	0.138		6.9	7.3	7.7	8.1	8.6	9.0	9.4
milking by hand	0.054		2.7	2.9	3.0	3.2	3.3	3.5	3.7
milking by machine	0.023		1.2	1.2	1.3	1.4	1.4	1.5	1.6
shoveling grain	0.085		4.3	4.5	4.8	5.0	5.3	5.5	5.8
Field hockey	0.134		6.7	7.1	7.5	7.9	8.3	8.7	9.1
Fishing	0.062		3.1	3.3	3.5	3.7	3.8	4.0	4.2
Food shopping (F)	0.062		3.1	3.3	3.5	3.7	3.8	4.0	4.2
Food shopping (M)	0.058		2.9	3.1	3.2	3.4	3.6	3.8	3.9
Football	0.132		6.6	7.0	7.4	7.8	8.2	8.6	9.0
Forestry									
ax chopping, fast	0.297		14.9	15.7	16.6	17.5	18.4	19.3	20.2
ax chopping, slow	0.085		4.3	4.5	4.8	5.0	5.3	5.5	5.8
barking trees	0.123		6.2	6.5	6.9	7.3	7.6	8.0	8.4
carrying logs	0.186		9.3	9.9	10.4	11.0	11.5	12.1	12.6
felling trees	0.132		6.6	7.0	7.4	7.8	8.2	8.6	9.0
hoeing	0.091		4.6	4.8	5.1	5.4	5.6	5.9	6.2
planting by hand	0.109		5.5	5.8	6.1	6.4	6.8	7.1	7.4
sawing by hand	0.122		6.1	6.5	6.8	7.2	7.6	7.9	8.3
sawing, power	0.075		3.8	4.0	4.2	4.4	4.7	4.9	5.1
stacking firewood	0.088		4.4	4.7	4.9	5.2	5.5	5.7	6.0
trimming trees	0.129		6.5	6.8	7.2	7.6	8.0	8.4	8.8
weeding	0.072		3.6	3.8	4.0	4.2	4.5	4.7	4.9
Furriery	0.083		4.2	4.4	4.6	4.9	5.1	5.4	5.6
Gardening									
digging	0.126		6.3	6.7	7.1	7.4	7.8	8.2	8.6
hedging	0.077		3.9	4.1	4.3	4.5	4.8	5.0	5.2
mowing	0.112		5.6	5.9	6.3	6.6	6.9	7.3	7.6
raking	0.054		2.7	2.9	3.0	3.2	3.3	3.5	3.7
Golf	0.085		4.3	4.5	4.8	5.0	5.3	5.5	5.8
Gymnastics	0.066		3.3	3.5	3.7	3.9	4.1	4.3	4.5
Horse-grooming	0.128		6.4	6.8	7.2	7.6	7.9	8.3	8.7
Horse-racing									
galloping	0.137		6.9	7.3	7.7	8.1	8.5	8.9	9.3

71 157	74 163	77 170	80 176	83 183	86 190	89 196	92 203	95 209	98 216
4.2	4.4	4.5	4.7	4.9	5.1	5.3	5.4	5.6	5.8
4.5	4.7	4.9	5.1	5.3	5.5	5.7	5.9	6.1	6.3
7.1	7.4	7.7	8.0	8.3	8.6	8.9	9.2	9.5	9.8
12.0	12.5	13.0	13.5	14.0	14.5	15.0	15.5	16.1	16.6
3.6	3.8	3.9	4.1	4.2	4.4	4.5	4.7	4.8	5.0
11.9	12.4	12.9	13.4	13.9	14.4	15.0	15.5	16.0	16.5
7.3	7.6	7.9	8.2	8.5	8.9	9.2	9.5	9.8	10.1
10.3	10.7	11.2	11.6	12.0	12.5	12.9	13.3	13.8	14.2
2.6	2.7	2.8	2.9	3.0	3.1	3.2	3.3	3.4	3.5
1.6	1.7	1.8	1.8	1.9	2.0	2.0	2.1	2.2	2.3
4.1	4.3	4.5	4.6	4.8	5.0	5.2	5.3	5.5	5.7
9.6	10.0	10.4	10.8	11.2	11.6	12.0	12.4	12.8	13.2
2.8	3.0	3.1	3.2	3.3	3.4	3.6	3.7	3.8	3.9
2.6	2.7	2.8	3.0	3.1	3.2	3.3	3.4	3.5	3.6
6.0	6.3	6.5	6.8	7.1	7.3	7.6	7.8	8.1	8.3
4.6	4.8	5.0	5.2	5.4	5.6	5.8	6.0	6.2	6.4
9.8	10.2	10.6	11.0	11.5	11.9	12.3	12.7	13.1	13.5
3.8	4.0	4.2	4.3	4.5	4.6	4.8	5.0	5.1	5.3
1.6	1.7	1.8	1.8	1.9	2.0	2.0	2.1	2.2	2.3
6.0	6.3	6.5	6.8	7.1	7.3	7.6	7.8	8.1	8.3
9.5	9.9	10.3	10.7	11.1	11.5	11.9	12.3	12.7	13.1
4.4	4.6	4.8	5.0	5.1	5.3	5.5	5.7	5.9	6.1
4.4	4.6	4.8	5.0	5.1	5.3	5.5	5.7	5.9	6.1
4.1	4.3	4.5	4.6	4.8	5.0	5.2	5.3	5.5	5.7
9.4	9.8	10.2	10.6	11.0	11.4	11.7	12.1	12.5	12.9
21.1	22.0	22.9	23.8	24.7	25.5	26.4	27.3	28.2	29.1
6.0	6.3	6.5	6.8	7.1	7.3	7.6	7.8	8.1	8.3
8.7	9.1	9.5	9.8	10.2	10.6	10.9	11.3	11.7	12.1
13.2	13.8	14.3	14.9	15.4	16.0	16.6	17.1	17.7	18.2
9.4	9.8	10.2	10.6	11.0	11.4	11.7	12.1	12.5	12.9
6.5	6.7	7.0	7.3	7.6	7.8	8.1	8.4	8.6	8.9
7.7	8.1	8.4	8.7	9.0	9.4	9.7	10.0	10.4	10.7
8.7	9.0	9.4	9.8	10.1	10.5	10.9	11.2	11.6	12.0
5.3	5.6	5.8	6.0	6.2	6.5	6.7	6.9	7.1	7.4
6.2	6.5	6.8	7.0	7.3	7.6	7.8	8.1	8.4	8.6
9.2	9.5	9.9	10.3	10.7	11.1	11.5	11.9	12.3	12.6
5.1	5.3	5.5	5.8	6.0	6.2	6.4	6.6	6.8	7.1
5.9	6.1	6.4	6.6	6.9	7.1	7.4	7.6	7.9	8.1
8.9	9.3	9.7	10.1	10.5	10.8	11.2	11.6	12.0	12.3
5.5	5.7	5.9	6.2	6.4	6.6	6.9	7.1	7.3	7.5
8.0	8.3	8.6	9.0	9.3	9.6	10.0	10.3	10.6	11.0
3.8	4.0	4.2	4.3	4.5	4.6	4.8	5.0	5.1	5.3
6.0	6.3	6.5	6.8	7.1	7.3	7.6	7.8	8.1	8.3
4.7	4.9	5.1	5.3	5.5	5.7	5.9	6.1	6.3	6.5
9.1	9.5	9.9	10.2	10.6	11.0	11.4	11.8	12.2	12.5
9.7	10.1	10.6	11.0	11.4	11.8	12.2	12.6	13.0	13.4

ACTIVITY	$kcal \cdot min^{-1} \cdot kg^{-1}$	kg 50 / lb 110	53 / 117	56 / 123	59 / 130	62 / 137	65 / 143	68 / 150
Horse-racing								
trotting	0.110	5.5	5.8	6.2	6.5	6.8	7.2	7.5
walking	0.041	2.1	2.2	2.3	2.4	2.5	2.7	2.8
Ironing (F)	0.033	1.7	1.7	1.8	1.9	2.0	2.1	2.2
Ironing (M)	0.064	3.2	3.4	3.6	3.8	4.0	4.2	4.4
Judo	0.195	9.8	10.3	10.9	11.5	12.1	12.7	13.3
Knitting, sewing (F)	0.022	1.1	1.2	1.2	1.3	1.4	1.4	1.5
Knitting, sewing (M)	0.023	1.2	1.2	1.3	1.4	1.4	1.5	1.6
Locksmith	0.057	2.9	3.0	3.2	3.4	3.5	3.7	3.9
Lying at ease	0.022	1.1	1.2	1.2	1.3	1.4	1.4	1.5
Machine-tooling								
machining	0.048	2.4	2.5	2.7	2.8	3.0	3.1	3.3
operating lathe	0.052	2.6	2.8	2.9	3.1	3.2	3.4	3.5
operating punch press	0.088	4.4	4.7	4.9	5.2	5.5	5.7	6.0
tapping and drilling	0.065	3.3	3.4	3.6	3.8	4.0	4.2	4.4
welding	0.052	2.6	2.8	2.9	3.1	3.2	3.4	3.5
working sheet metal	0.048	2.4	2.5	2.7	2.8	3.0	3.1	3.3
Marching, rapid	0.142	7.1	7.5	8.0	8.4	8.8	9.2	9.7
Mopping floor (F)	0.062	3.1	3.3	3.5	3.7	3.8	4.0	4.2
Mopping floor (M)	0.058	2.9	3.1	3.2	3.4	3.6	3.8	3.9
Music playing								
accordion (sitting)	0.032	1.6	1.7	1.8	1.9	2.0	2.1	2.2
cello (sitting)	0.041	2.1	2.2	2.3	2.4	2.5	2.7	2.8
conducting	0.039	2.0	2.1	2.2	2.3	2.4	2.5	2.7
drums (sitting)	0.066	3.3	3.5	3.7	3.9	4.1	4.3	4.5
flute (sitting)	0.035	1.8	1.9	2.0	2.1	2.2	2.3	2.4
horn (sitting)	0.029	1.5	1.5	1.6	1.7	1.8	1.9	2.0
organ (sitting)	0.053	2.7	2.8	3.0	3.1	3.3	3.4	3.6
piano (sitting)	0.040	2.0	2.1	2.2	2.4	2.5	2.6	2.7
trumpet (standing)	0.031	1.6	1.6	1.7	1.8	1.9	2.0	2.1
violin (sitting)	0.045	2.3	2.4	2.5	2.7	2.8	2.9	3.1
woodwind (sitting)	0.032	1.6	1.7	1.8	1.9	2.0	2.1	2.2
Painting, inside	0.034	1.7	1.8	1.9	2.0	2.1	2.2	2.3
Painting, outside	0.077	3.9	4.1	4.3	4.5	4.8	5.0	5.2
Planting seedlings	0.070	3.5	3.7	3.9	4.1	4.3	4.6	4.8
Plastering	0.078	3.9	4.1	4.4	4.6	4.8	5.1	5.3
Printing	0.035	1.8	1.9	2.0	2.1	2.2	2.3	2.4
Running, cross-country	0.163	8.2	8.6	9.1	9.6	10.1	10.6	11.1
Running, horizontal								
11 min, 30 s per mile	0.135	6.8	7.2	7.6	8.0	8.4	8.8	9.2
9 min per mile	0.193	9.7	10.2	10.8	11.4	12.0	12.5	13.1
8 min per mile	0.208	10.8	11.3	11.9	12.5	13.1	13.6	14.2
7 min per mile	0.228	12.2	12.7	13.3	13.9	14.5	15.0	15.6
6 min per mile	0.252	13.9	14.4	15.0	15.6	16.2	16.7	17.3
5 min, 30 s per mile	0.289	14.5	15.3	16.2	17.1	17.9	18.8	19.7
Scraping paint	0.063	3.2	3.3	3.5	3.7	3.9	4.1	4.3
Scrubbing floors (F)	0.109	5.5	5.8	6.1	6.4	6.8	7.1	7.4
Scrubbing floors (M)	0.108	5.4	5.7	6.0	6.4	6.7	7.0	7.3
Shoe repair, general	0.045	2.3	2.4	2.5	2.7	2.8	2.9	3.1

71 157	74 163	77 170	80 176	83 183	86 190	89 196	92 203	95 209	98 216
7.8	8.1	8.5	8.8	9.1	9.5	9.8	10.1	10.5	10.8
2.9	3.0	3.2	3.3	3.4	3.5	3.6	3.8	3.9	4.0
2.3	2.4	2.5	2.6	2.7	2.8	2.9	3.0	3.1	3.2
4.5	4.7	4.9	5.1	5.3	5.5	5.7	5.9	6.1	6.3
13.8	14.4	15.0	15.6	16.2	16.8	17.4	17.9	18.5	19.1
1.6	1.6	1.7	1.8	1.8	1.9	2.0	2.0	2.1	2.2
1.6	1.7	1.8	1.8	1.9	2.0	2.0	2.1	2.2	2.3
4.0	4.2	4.4	4.6	4.7	4.9	5.1	5.2	5.4	5.6
1.6	1.6	1.7	1.8	1.8	1.9	2.0	2.0	2.1	2.2
3.4	3.6	3.7	3.8	4.0	4.1	4.3	4.4	4.6	4.7
3.7	3.8	4.0	4.2	4.3	4.5	4.6	4.8	4.9	5.1
6.2	6.5	6.8	7.0	7.3	7.6	7.8	8.1	8.4	8.6
4.6	4.8	5.0	5.2	5.4	5.6	5.8	6.0	6.2	6.4
3.7	3.8	4.0	4.2	4.3	4.5	4.6	4.8	4.9	5.1
3.4	3.6	3.7	3.8	4.0	4.1	4.3	4.4	4.6	4.7
10.1	10.5	10.9	11.4	11.8	12.2	12.6	13.1	13.5	13.9
4.4	4.6	4.8	5.0	5.1	5.3	5.5	5.7	5.9	6.1
4.1	4.3	4.5	4.6	4.8	5.0	5.2	5.	5.5	5.7
2.3	2.4	2.5	2.6	2.7	2.8	2.8	2.9	3.0	3.1
2.9	3.0	3.2	3.3	3.4	3.5	3.6	3.8	3.9	4.0
2.8	2.9	3.0	3.1	3.2	3.4	3.5	3.6	3.7	3.8
4.7	4.9	5.1	5.3	5.5	5.7	5.9	6.1	6.3	6.6
2.5	2.6	2.7	2.8	2.9	3.0	3.1	3.2	3.3	3.4
2.1	2.1	2.2	2.3	2.4	2.5	2.6	2.7	2.8	2.8
3.8	3.9	4.1	4.2	4.4	4.6	4.7	4.9	5.0	5.2
2.8	3.0	3.1	3.2	3.3	3.4	3.6	3.7	3.8	3.9
2.2	2.3	2.4	2.5	2.6	2.7	2.8	2.9	2.9	3.0
3.2	3.3	3.5	3.6	3.7	3.9	4.0	4.1	4.3	4.4
2.3	2.4	2.5	2.6	2.7	2.8	2.8	2.9	3.0	3.1
2.4	2.5	2.6	2.7	2.8	2.9	3.0	3.1	3.2	3.3
5.5	5.7	5.9	6.2	6.4	6.6	6.9	7.1	7.3	7.5
5.0	5.2	5.4	5.6	5.8	6.0	6.2	6.4	6.7	6.9
5.5	5.8	6.0	6.2	6.5	6.7	6.9	7.2	7.4	7.6
2.5	2.6	2.7	2.8	2.9	3.0	3.1	3.2	3.3	3.4
11.6	12.1	12.6	13.0	13.5	14.0	14.5	15.0	15.5	16.0
9.6	10.0	10.5	10.9	11.3	11.7	12.1	12.5	12.9	13.3
13.7	14.3	14.9	15.4	16.0	16.6	17.2	17.8	18.3	18.9
14.8	15.4	16.0	16.5	17.1	17.7	18.3	18.9	19.4	20.0
16.2	16.8	17.4	17.9	18.5	19.1	19.7	20.3	20.8	21.4
17.9	18.5	19.1	19.6	20.2	20.8	21.4	22.0	22.5	23.1
20.5	21.4	22.3	23.1	24.0	24.9	25.7	26.6	27.5	28.3
4.5	4.7	4.9	5.0	5.2	5.4	5.6	5.8	6.0	6.2
7.7	8.1	8.4	8.7	9.0	9.4	9.7	10.0	10.4	10.7
7.7	8.0	8.3	8.6	9.0	9.3	9.6	9.9	10.3	10.6
3.2	3.3	3.5	3.6	3.7	3.9	4.0	4.1	4.3	4.4

ACTIVITY	$kcal \cdot min^{-1} \cdot kg^{-1}$	kg 50 / lb 110	53 / 117	56 / 123	59 / 130	62 / 137	65 / 143	68 / 150
Sitting quietly	0.021	1.1	1.1	1.2	1.2	1.3	1.4	1.4
Skiing, hard snow								
level, moderate speed	0.119	6.0	6.3	6.7	7.0	7.4	7.7	8.1
level, walking	0.143	7.2	7.6	8.0	8.4	8.9	9.3	9.7
uphill, maximum speed	0.274	13.7	14.5	15.3	16.2	17.0	17.8	18.6
Skiing, soft snow								
leisure (F)	0.111	4.9	5.2	5.5	5.8	6.1	6.4	6.7
leisure (M)	0.098	5.6	5.9	6.2	6.5	6.9	7.2	7.5
Skindiving, as frogman								
considerable motion	0.276	13.8	14.6	15.5	16.3	17.1	17.9	18.8
moderate motion	0.206	10.3	10.9	11.5	12.2	12.8	13.4	14.0
Snowshoeing, soft snow	0.166	8.3	8.8	9.3	9.8	10.3	10.8	11.3
Squash	0.212	10.6	11.2	11.9	12.5	13.1	13.8	14.4
Standing quietly (F)	0.025	1.3	1.3	1.4	1.5	1.6	1.6	1.7
Standing quietly (M)	0.027	1.4	1.4	1.5	1.6	1.7	1.8	1.8
Steel mill, working in								
fettling	0.089	4.5	4.7	5.0	5.3	5.5	5.8	6.1
forging	0.100	5.0	5.3	5.6	5.9	6.2	6.5	6.8
hand rolling	0.137	6.9	7.3	7.7	8.1	8.5	8.9	9.3
merchant mill rolling	0.145	7.3	7.7	8.1	8.6	9.0	9.4	9.9
removing slag	0.178	8.9	9.4	10.0	10.5	11.0	11.6	12.1
tending furnace	0.126	6.3	6.7	7.1	7.4	7.8	8.2	8.6
tipping molds	0.092	4.6	4.9	5.2	5.4	5.7	6.0	6.3
Stock clerking	0.054	2.7	2.9	3.0	3.2	3.3	3.5	3.7
Swimming								
backstroke	0.169	8.5	9.0	9.5	10.0	10.5	11.0	11.5
breast stroke	0.162	8.1	8.6	9.1	9.6	10.0	10.5	11.0
crawl, fast	0.156	7.8	8.3	8.7	9.2	9.7	10.1	10.6
crawl, slow	0.128	6.4	6.8	7.2	7.6	7.9	8.3	8.7
side stroke	0.122	6.1	6.5	6.8	7.2	7.6	7.9	8.3
treading, fast	0.170	8.5	9.0	9.5	10.0	10.5	11.1	11.6
treading, normal	0.062	3.1	3.3	3.5	3.7	3.8	4.0	4.2
Table tennis	0.068	3.4	3.6	3.8	4.0	4.2	4.4	4.6
Tailoring								
cutting	0.041	2.1	2.2	2.3	2.4	2.5	2.7	2.8
hand-sewing	0.032	1.6	1.7	1.8	1.9	2.0	2.1	2.2
machine-sewing	0.045	2.3	2.4	2.5	2.7	2.8	2.9	3.1
pressing	0.062	3.1	3.3	3.5	3.7	3.8	4.0	4.2
Tennis	0.109	5.5	5.8	6.1	6.4	6.8	7.1	7.4
Typing								
electric	0.027	1.4	1.4	1.5	1.6	1.7	1.8	1.8
manual	0.031	1.6	1.6	1.7	1.8	1.9	2.0	2.1
Volleyball	0.050	2.5	2.7	2.8	3.0	3.1	3.3	3.4
Walking, normal pace								
asphalt road	0.080	4.0	4.2	4.5	4.7	5.0	5.2	5.4
fields and hillsides	0.082	4.1	4.3	4.6	4.8	5.1	5.3	5.6
grass track	0.081	4.1	4.3	4.5	4.8	5.0	5.3	5.5
plowed field	0.077	3.9	4.1	4.3	4.5	4.8	5.0	5.2
Wallpapering	0.048	2.4	2.5	2.7	2.8	3.0	3.1	3.3
Watch repairing	0.025	1.3	1.3	1.4	1.5	1.6	1.6	1.7
Window cleaning (F)	0.059	3.0	3.1	3.3	3.5	3.7	3.8	4.0
Window cleaning (M)	0.058	2.9	3.1	3.2	3.4	3.6	3.8	3.9
Writing (sitting)	0.029	1.5	1.5	1.6	1.7	1.8	1.9	2.0

| 71 | 74 | 77 | 80 | 83 | 86 | 89 | 92 | 95 | 98 |
157	163	170	176	183	190	196	203	209	216
1.5	1.6	1.6	1.7	1.7	1.8	1.9	1.9	2.0	2.1
8.4	8.8	9.2	9.5	9.9	10.2	10.6	10.9	11.3	11.7
10.2	10.6	11.0	11.4	11.9	12.3	12.7	13.2	13.6	14.0
19.5	20.3	21.1	21.9	22.7	23.6	24.4	25.2	26.0	26.9
7.0	7.3	7.5	7.8	8.1	8.4	8.7	9.0	9.3	9.6
7.9	8.2	8.5	8.9	9.2	9.5	9.9	10.2	10.5	10.9
19.6	20.4	21.3	22.1	22.9	23.7	24.6	25.4	26.2	27.0
14.6	15.2	15.9	16.5	17.1	17.7	18.3	19.0	19.6	20.2
11.8	12.3	12.8	13.3	13.8	14.3	14.8	15.3	15.8	16.3
15.1	15.7	16.3	17.0	17.6	18.2	18.9	19.5	20.1	20.8
1.8	1.9	1.9	2.0	2.1	2.2	2.2	2.3	2.4	2.5
1.9	2.0	2.1	2.2	2.2	2.3	2.4	2.5	2.6	2.6
6.3	6.6	6.9	7.1	7.4	7.7	7.9	8.2	8.5	8.7
7.1	7.4	7.7	8.0	8.3	8.6	8.9	9.2	9.5	9.8
9.7	10.1	10.6	11.0	11.4	11.8	12.2	12.6	13.0	13.4
10.3	10.7	11.2	11.6	12.0	12.5	12.9	13.3	13.8	14.2
12.6	13.2	13.7	14.2	14.8	15.3	15.8	16.4	16.9	17.4
8.9	9.3	9.7	10.1	10.5	10.8	11.2	11.6	12.0	12.3
6.5	6.8	7.1	7.4	7.6	7.9	8.2	8.5	8.7	9.0
3.8	4.0	4.2	4.3	4.5	4.6	4.8	5.0	5.1	5.3
12.0	12.5	13.0	13.5	14.0	14.5	15.0	15.5	16.1	16.6
11.5	12.0	12.5	13.0	13.4	13.9	14.4	14.9	15.4	15.9
11.1	11.5	12.0	12.5	12.9	13.4	13.9	14.4	14.8	15.3
9.1	9.5	9.9	10.2	10.6	11.0	11.4	11.8	12.2	12.5
8.7	9.0	9.4	9.8	10.1	10.5	10.9	11.2	11.6	12.0
12.1	12.6	13.1	13.6	14.1	14.6	15.1	15.6	16.2	16.7
4.4	4.6	4.8	5.0	5.1	5.3	5.5	5.7	5.9	6.1
4.8	5.0	5.2	5.4	5.6	5.8	6.1	6.3	6.5	6.7
2.9	3.0	3.2	3.3	3.4	3.5	3.6	3.8	3.9	4.0
2.3	2.4	2.5	2.6	2.7	2.8	2.8	2.9	3.0	3.1
3.2	3.3	3.5	3.6	3.7	3.9	4.0	4.1	4.3	4.4
4.4	4.6	4.8	5.0	5.1	5.3	5.5	5.7	5.9	6.1
7.7	8.1	8.4	8.7	9.0	9.4	9.7	10.0	10.4	10.7
1.9	2.0	2.1	2.2	2.2	2.3	2.4	2.5	2.6	2.6
2.2	2.3	2.4	2.5	2.6	2.7	2.8	2.9	2.9	3.0
3.6	3.7	3.9	4.0	4.2	4.3	4.5	4.6	4.8	4.9
5.7	5.9	6.2	6.4	6.6	6.9	7.1	7.4	7.6	7.8
5.8	6.1	6.3	6.6	6.8	7.1	7.3	7.5	7.8	8.0
5.8	6.0	6.2	6.5	6.7	7.0	7.2	7.5	7.7	7.9
5.5	5.7	5.9	6.2	6.4	6.6	6.9	7.1	7.3	7.5
3.4	3.6	3.7	3.8	4.0	4.1	4.3	4.4	4.6	4.7
1.8	1.9	1.9	2.0	2.1	2.2	2.2	2.3	2.4	2.5
4.2	4.4	4.5	4.7	4.9	5.1	5.3	5.4	5.6	5.8
4.1	4.3	4.5	4.6	4.8	5.0	5.2	5.3	5.5	5.7
2.1	2.1	2.2	2.3	2.4	2.5	2.6	2.7	2.8	2.8

APPENDIX II: NUTRITION SCOREBOARD

VEGETABLES

Most vegetables are great sources of vitamins—especially A and C—and minerals and usually taste best either raw or just lightly cooked. Try a new vegetable today!

spinach, fresh	2 cups, raw	91
collard greens, fresh	½ cup, cooked	90
sweet potato	1 med., baked	82
potato	1 med., baked	71
kale, fresh	½ cup, cooked	71
winter squash (acorn, butternut)	½ cup, baked	70
broccoli, fresh	½ cup, cooked	68
asparagus, fresh	½ cup, cooked	67
spinach, frozen	½ cup, cooked	65
mixed vegetables, frozen	½ cup, cooked	63
broccoli, frozen	½ cup, cooked	59
brussel sprouts, fresh	½ cup, cooked	58
tomato	1 medium	56
rutabaga	½ cup, cooked	54
carrot	1 medium	48
green peas, frozen	1/2 cup, cooked	45
green pepper	1/2 cup	44
sweet corn, fresh (on-the-cob)	1 ear, cooked	41
cauliflower, fresh	½ cup, raw	36
cabbage, chopped	1 cup, raw	36
okra	½ cup, cooked	34
yellow corn, canned[1]	½ cup, drained	34
sweet peas, canned[1]	½ cup, drained	33
asparagus, canned[1]	½ cup, cooked	23
artichoke, fresh	½ bud	23
green beans, fresh	½ cup, cooked	22
summer squash (zucchini)	½ cup, cooked	22
turnips	½ cup, cooked	21
bean sprouts	½ cup	18
eggplant	½ cup, cooked	18
lettuce, romaine	1 cup	17
green beans, canned[1]	½ cup, drained	17
sauerkraut[1]	½ cup, drained	14
onion, chopped	¼ cup, raw	12
lettuce, iceberg	1 cup	11
mushrooms, fresh	¼ cup, raw	9
avocado[2]	½ medium	6
cucumber	5 slices	6

[1] Canned vegetables are all high in salt.

[2] Avocado is the only high-fat vegetable.

FRUITS

Fruits can give you, naturally, all the sweetness you want, plus fiber and a wide variety of vitamins and minerals, especially vitamins A and C.

watermelon	10"x1" slice	68
papaya	½ medium	60
cantaloupe	¼ medium	60
mango	½ medium	52
orange	1 medium	49
grapefruit	½ medium	42
banana	1 medium	36
honeydew melon	7"x2" slice	35
strawberries	½ cup	34
pear	1 medium	29
raspberries	½ cup	27
peach	1 medium	26
prunes, uncooked	3 medium	26
tangerine	1 medium	26
apple	1 medium	23
blueberries	½ cup	21
pineapple, fresh	½ cup	18
cherries	½ cup	17
pomegranate	½ fruit	14
plum, red	1 medium	12
grapes	½ cup	10

BEVERAGES

Most beverages made from fruits and vegetables are high in vitamins A and C and natural sugars; they also contain modest amounts of other vitamins and minerals. While some low-scoring beverages may be fortified with one or two vitamins, they are all high in added sugar (or contain saccharin). Finally, don't forget water!

carrot juice	6 oz.	48
orange juice, unsweetened	6 oz.	47
tomato juice	6 oz.	36
grapefruit juice, unsweetened	6 oz.	36
V-8 juice	6 oz.	26
apple juice	6 oz.	23
grape juice, frozen	6 oz.	15
pineapple-grapefruit juice	6 oz.	11
coffee or tea[1]	6 oz.	0
Tab, other diet sodas[2]	12 oz., 1 can	−1
Awake	6 oz.	−3
Cranberry Juice Cocktail	6 oz.	−6
Tang	6 oz.	−9
Hawaiian Punch	6 oz.	−13
Hi-C	6 oz.	−15
Welchade Grape Drink	6 oz.	−19
lemonade	6 oz.	−20
Kool-Aid, presweetened	6 oz.	−21
Gatorade	12 oz., 1 can	−34
Coca-Cola, other sodas[1]	12 oz., 1 can	−55

[1] Scientific studies indicate that moderate amounts of caffeine can cause birth defects and other reproductive problems. Pregnant women should minimize their intake of coffee, tea, and caffeine-containing soft drinks.

[2] Diet sodas contain saccharin, an artificial sweetener that causes cancer in animals, and probably in humans. The more saccharin consumed, the greater the risk.

HOW TO USE THIS CHART

The charts on this poster indicate the relative nutritional values of many common foods. In general, comparisons should be made within each category: the higher the score, the more nutritious the food. Choose foods that are near the tops of the charts; eat less of the foods that have negative values or are near the bottoms. Small differences in ratings (e.g. 24 vs. 26) are not significant.

Eat a varied diet composed mainly of grains and grain products (especially whole grains), fresh vegetables and fruits, poultry and fish, lowfat dairy products, lean meats, dried beans, and nuts. Eat fewer foods that are high in fat, salt, sugar, and cholesterol.

Foods have been given points for their content of protein, dietary fiber, naturally-occurring sugars and starch, polyunsaturated fat, four vitamins (*A, C, riboflavin (B-2), and niacin (B-3)*), and two minerals (*iron and calcium*). Points were deducted for total fat content, saturated and monounsaturated fat, cholesterol, sodium, and added sugars.

The formulas used to score foods reflect current scientific beliefs about nutrition and health. A diet high in saturated fat and cholesterol greatly increases the risk of coronary heart disease. Diets high in any kind of fat—saturated or unsaturated—are likely to increase the risk of bowel and breast cancers. Too much salt (*sodium*) can promote high blood pressure, which increases the risk of heart attack and stroke. Sugar promotes tooth decay and obesity, while pushing nutritious foods out of one's diet.

The single most beneficial dietary change for most people would be to replace fatty foods with foods rich in starch and dietary fiber (potatoes, whole wheat bread, brown rice, dried beans, etc.).

Ratings listed are for average-size servings. Adjust the score proportionately for larger or smaller portions.

Ratings of different items can be added together. For instance, a tuna-fish sandwich would have a score of 112: *tuna, 75; whole wheat bread, 55; 1 Tbsp. mayonnaise, -18.* If a food is not listed, use the rating of a similar food.

While the ratings may be added, there is no magic goal to aim for each day. A healthy diet must be moderate, varied, and enjoyable.

BON APPETIT!

DAIRY

The best dairy foods are the lowfat milks, yogurts, and cottage cheeses. While all dairy foods are good sources of protein, calcium, and riboflavin, the lower-scoring foods are high in saturated fat and sodium.

yogurt, lowfat, plain	8 oz., 1 cup	64
skim milk	8 oz.	55
buttermilk, 1% fat	8 oz.	46
lowfat milk, 2% fat	8 oz.	43
soymilk	8 oz.	33
cottage cheese, 1% fat	½ cup	30
whole milk	8 oz.	28
chocolate milk, 2% fat	8 oz.	27
ricotta cheese, part skim	½ cup	26
lowfat American cheese	2 oz.	26
mozzarella cheese, part skim	2 oz.	19
cottage cheese, 4% fat	2 oz.	17
yogurt, whole milk, plain	8 oz., 1 cup	15
Swiss cheese	2 oz.	13
yogurt, lowfat, fruit	8 oz., 1 cup	10
ricotta cheese, whole milk	½ cup	−1
mozzarella cheese, whole milk	2 oz.	−1
cheddar cheese	2 oz.	−10
cream cheese	½ oz., 1 cub. in.	−11
American cheese	2 oz.	−18

POULTRY, FISH, MEAT & EGGS

Lower-scoring foods tend to be high in calories, cholesterol (eggs), fat (red meat), or sodium (processed meats). The foods near the top are excellent sources of iron, protein, and other nutrients. See footnote[1] below for information about liver, an unusual food that rates special consideration. These foods are most nutritious when baked, broiled, or poached instead of fried.

Red meat scores are for cooked, semi-trimmed cuts. If more than half the removable fat is trimmed away, scores would improve; if less than half is removed, the scores would fall.

tuna, waterpack	3 oz.	75
lobster, cooked meat	3 oz.	72
chicken, roasted, skinless	3 oz.	68
salmon, pink, fillet	3 oz.	67
turkey, roasted	3 oz.	62
flounder, baked	3 oz.	54
scallops, steamed	3 oz.	52
salmon, sockeye red, canned	3 oz.	52
shrimp, steamed	3 oz.	52
round steak	3 oz.	51
cod, broiled	3 oz.	50
crabs, steamed meat	3 oz. (1 cup)	46
veal cutlet, broiled	3 oz.	44
clams, raw or steamed	5 clams (2.5 oz.)	43
chicken, roasted w/skin	3 oz.	42
tuna, oilpack, drained	3 oz.	40
leg of lamb	3 oz.	34
shrimp, fried, breaded	3 oz.	31
ham, baked[2]	3 oz.	28
chicken, fried, breaded	2 oz., 1 thigh	27
rump roast	3 oz.	26
pork chop, baked	3 oz.	25
Canadian style bacon[2]	2 slices (2 oz.)	21
sirloin steak	3 oz.	17
hamburger, 20% fat, lean	3 oz.	14
ham, smoked[2]	2 slices (2 oz.)	12
egg white	1 large egg white	11
hamburger, 25% fat, regular	3 oz.	−4
bacon[2]	2 slices (½ oz.)	−5
egg	1 large	−7
chicken hot dog, lowfat[2]	1 (1.6 oz.)	−7
hard salami	2 oz.	−18
pork sausage	3 links (2 oz.)	−19
hot dog[2]	1 (1.6 oz.)	−20
beef bologna[2]	2 slices (2 oz.)	−26
luncheon meat[2]	2 slices (2 oz.)	−33
Spam[2]	3 oz.	−35

[1] Liver is rich in iron, protein, trace minerals and numerous vitamins, and is low in fat. However, it is high in cholesterol and may be contaminated with pollutants. Eat liver only occasionally.

[2] These meats contain sodium nitrite, an additive that can react with other chemicals to form a cancer-causing nitrosamine. The more nitrite consumed, the greater the risk.

GRAIN FOODS

Contrary to a widespread myth, starchy grain foods are not fattening. Most people would do well to eat more grain foods in place of meat. Grains, especially whole grains, are a nicely-balanced, lowfat source of carbohydrates, vitamins, minerals, and protein.

bulghur (cracked wheat)	½ cup, cooked	77
whole wheat pita (Syrian) bread	1 pouch	73
whole wheat bread	2 slices	55
millet	½ cup, cooked	52
brown rice	½ cup, cooked	47
rye bread	2 slices	46
white bread, enriched	2 slices	45
white rice, enriched	½ cup, cooked	45
pearled barley	½ cup, cooked	42
cornbread	2" square	38
hamburger/hotdog roll, enriched	1	36
instant white rice, enriched	½ cup, cooked	36
spaghetti or macaroni, enriched	½ cup, cooked	32
pancakes, buckwheat (mix)	four 4" cakes	31
oatmeal	½ cup, cooked	30
wheat germ	2 Tbsp.	24
hominy grits	½ cup, cooked	23

BEANS, NUTS, & SEEDS

Beans, nuts, and seeds are excellent sources of dietary fiber, protein, vitamins, and minerals. While beans are generally low in fat, peanuts and most nuts and seeds are high in both fat and calories.

black beans	½ cup, cooked	93
chickpeas (garbanzo beans)	½ cup, cooked	90
lima beans	½ cup, cooked	73
navy beans	½ cup, cooked	61
lentils	½ cup, cooked	57
kidney beans	½ cup, cooked	56
split peas	½ cup, cooked	51
black-eyed peas	½ cup, cooked	49
soybeans	½ cup, cooked	46
tofu (bean curd)	1 piece, (4 oz.), 2½"x2¾"x1"	31
sunflower seeds, hulled	1 oz.	24
almonds, shelled	1 oz.	18
peanuts, roasted	1 oz.	11
cashews	1 oz.	7
peanut butter	2 Tbsp.	5
English walnuts	1 oz.	3
sesame seeds	1 oz.	2

CONDIMENTS

Go easy on the condiments, which can easily add unwanted salt, fat, or sugar to your diet.

tomato sauce	¼ cup	13
molasses	1 tsp.	2
low-calorie Italian dressing	1 Tbsp.	0
catsup	1 Tbsp.	−1
soy sauce	1 tsp.	−2
cream, half and half	1 Tbsp.	−2
imitation mayonnaise	1 tsp.	−3
diet margarine	1 tsp.	−3
safflower oil	1 tsp.	−3
whipped cream	1 Tbsp.	−3
salt	1/4 tsp.	−4
sour cream	1 Tbsp.	−4
coffee whitener	1 Tbsp.	−5
soft margarine	1 pat.	−5
Cool Whip	1 Tbsp.	−5
jelly	1 tsp.	−6
mayonnaise	1 tsp.	−6
pancake syrup	1 Tbsp.	−6
margarine, stick	1 pat	−6
French salad dressing	1 Tbsp.	−6
cream, light	1 Tbsp.	−6
sugar	1 tsp.	−6
honey[1]	1 tsp.	−7
cranberry sauce	1 Tbsp.	−7
butter	1 pat	−13

[1] Honey is essentially an unprocessed sugar and contains insignificant amounts of nutrients. Both honey and sugar promote tooth decay.

SNACKS

Try to keep nutritious snacks—hot or cold, crisp or mushy—around your house and workplace so you won't be tempted to eat junk foods. Most packaged chips and similar snacks add salt, unwanted calories, and questionable preservatives to your diet. Crisp raw vegetables, fresh fruit, and moderate amounts of nuts and seeds all make great snacks!

carrot	1 medium	48
green pepper	½ cup	44
dried apricots[1]	2 medium	31
raisins[1]	1 box (1.5 oz.)	28
soynuts, salted	1 oz.	28
apple	1 medium	23
pretzels, 3-ringed	3 pretzels	19
popcorn, plain	2 cups	19
celery	four 5" pieces	17
Ry-Krisps	2 triple crackers	17
potato chips	1 oz.	15
corn chips	1 oz.	13
graham crackers	2 crackers, 2½" square	12
saltine crackers	4 crackers	10
jumbo peanuts (in the shell)	10	9
popcorn, butter and salt	2 cups	6
Cheez-its	10 crackers	5
Pringles potato chips	1 oz.	4
dill pickle	1 medium	−3
sugar wafers	2	−3
Popsicle	1	−27
marshmallows	4	−28
Hostess Twinkies	1 package	−34
Hunts Vanilla Snackpack Pudding	1 can, 5 oz.	−34
jellybeans	10	−38
Hershey's milk chocolate	1 bar (1.5 oz.)	−42

[1] Go easy on the dried fruits! Their natural sugars are sticky and can promote tooth decay.

DESSERTS

Most desserts are high in fat, sugar and calories. Next time, try fresh fruit for a change!

cantaloupe	¼ medium	60
strawberries	½ cup	34
applesauce, unsweetened	½ cup	17
pineapple, canned in juice	½ cup	17
blueberry muffin	1 muffin	8
vanilla ice milk	½ cup	7
frozen yogurt, lowfat, vanilla	½ cup	3
frozen yogurt, lowfat, fruit	½ cup	−1
angelfood cake	1 med. slice	−1
orange sherbet	½ cup	−2
chocolate pudding	½ cup	−7
pears, heavy syrup	½ cup	−8
sponge cake	1 med. slice	−10
peaches, heavy syrup	½ cup	−10
applesauce, sweetened	½ cup	−10
brownies w/nuts	1¾" square	−12
apple pie alamode	med. slice with small scoop ice cream	−15
cupcake, plain	1	−16
pound cake, old-fashioned	1 med. slice	−18
vanilla ice cream	½ cup	−22
Jell-O, flavored	½ cup	−26
Sara Lee chocolate cake, frozen	1 med. slice	−27
chocolate eclair	1	−30

BREAKFAST CEREALS

The best cereals are whole grain and relatively unprocessed. Among processed cereals look for whole grain, low sugar content, and no artificial colorings and flavorings. Companies have fortified many cereals with vitamins and minerals in part to distract attention from the products' high sugar content. Since the Nutrition Scoreboard *system is not designed to handle fortifications equivalent to vitamin pills, figures below indicate percentage of sugar by weight (including all naturally-occurring sugars).* Better choices are indicated in* **bold-face**.

	% sugar by weight		% sugar by weight
Wheat germ	0	Frosted Mini-Wheats	26
Oatmeal	0	C.W. Post	29
Farina	0	Raisin Bran	30
Wheatena	0	Golden Grahams	30
Puffed wheat or rice	0	Cocoa Puffs	33
Shredded Wheat	1	Trix	36
Cheerios	3	Honey Comb	37
Wheat-, Corn-, Rice-Chex	4	Alpha Bits	38
Kix	5	Count Chocula	40
Corn Flakes	5	Cap'n Crunch	40
Special K	5	Crazy Cow	40
Grapenuts	7	Sugar Frosted Flakes	41
Rice Krispies	8	Lucky Charms	42
Wheaties; Total	8	Cocoa-, Fruity Pebbles	43
Concentrate	9	Cookie Crisp, vanilla	44
Product 19	10	Frankenberry	44
40% Bran	13	Super Sugar Crisp	46
Life	16	Froot Loops	48
All Bran	19	Apple Jacks	55
100% Bran	21	Sugar Smacks	56
Quaker 100% Natural Cereal	21		

Most cereal boxes now declare "grams of added sugar" on their side panels. Next time, do your teeth a favor and compare!

*Figures from U.S. Dept. Agriculture.

The Center for Science in the Public Interest

The Center for Science in the Public Interest seeks to improve the public's health by offering reliable nutrition information and working for better food and health policies. CSPI is a non-profit group. Send for a free list of publications and membership information.

What You Can Do

If you would like the government to promote better nutrition, write to your elected officials, the Commissioner of FDA (Rockville, Md. 20857), and the Secretary of Agriculture (Washington D.C. 20250).

INDEX